D0146153

# Ultrasound and the Fetal Heart

PROGRESS IN OBSTETRIC
AND GYNECOLOGICAL
SONOGRAPHY SERIES

SERIES EDITOR: ASIM KURJAK

# Ultrasound and the Fetal Heart

Edited by

## J. W. WLADIMIROFF and G. PILU

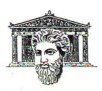

**The Parthenon Publishing Group**

International Publishers in Medicine, Science & Technology

NEW YORK                                                    LONDON

7.97

**Library of Congress Cataloging-in-Publication Data**

Ultrasound and the fetal heart/edited by J. Wladimiroff and G. Pilu.

  p. cm.—(Progress in obstetric and gynecological sonography series)

  Includes bibliographical references and index.
  ISBN 1-85070-617-4

  1. Fetal heart—Ultrasonic imaging.   2. Fetal heart—Abnormalities.   I. Wladimiroff. Juriy W. II. Pilu, G. III. Series.

  [DNLM:   1. Ultrasonography. Prenatal—methods.   2. Heart Defects. Congenital—ultrasonography.   3. Fetal Heart—ultrasonography.   WQ 209 U4675 1996]
RG628.3.E34U48 1996
618.3'26107543—dc20
DNLM/DLC
for Library of Congress                    96-30590
                                                          CIP


**British Library Cataloguing in Publication Data**

Ultrasound and the fetal heart.—(Progress in obstetric and gynecological sonography series)

  1. Fetal heart—Imaging   2. Echo cardiography
  I. Wladimiroff, Juriy W.   II. Pilu, G.
  618.3'2'07543

  ISBN 1-85070-617-4

Published in North America by
The Parthenon Publishing Group Inc.
One Blue Hill Plaza
Pearl River
New York 10965, USA


Published in the UK and Europe by
The Parthenon Publishing Group Limited
Casterton Hall, Carnforth
Lancs. LA6 2LA, UK

Copyright © 1996 Parthenon Publishing Group

First published 1996

*No part of this publication may be reproduced in any form without permission from the publishers, except for the quotation of brief passages for the purpose of review*

Typeset by AMA Graphics Ltd., Preston, Lancashire, UK
Printed and bound by Butler & Tanner Ltd., Frome and London

# Contents

# List of principal contributors

**J. I. Brenner**
Division of Pediatric Cardiology
22 S. Greene Street
Baltimore MD 21201
USA

**M. L. A. Broekhuizen**
Department of Obstetrics and Gynecology
University Hospital Rotterdam
Dr Molewaterplein 40
3015 GD Rotterdam
The Netherlands

**E. Buskens**
Department of Pediatrics
Division of Pediatric Cardiology
Sophia Children's Hospital
Dr Molewaterplein 60
3015 GJ Rotterdam
*and*
Department of Epidemiology and Biostatistics
Erasmus University Medical School Rotterdam
Dr Molewaterplein 50
3015 GJ Rotterdam
The Netherlands

**J. A. Copel**
Department of Obstetrics and Gynecology
Yale University School of Medicine
PO Box 208063
New Haven CT 06520-8063
USA

**U. Gembruch**
Division of Prenatal Medicine
Department of Obstetrics and Gynecology
Medical University of Lübeck
D-23538 Lübeck
Germany

**A. C. Gittenberger-de Groot**
Department of Anatomy and Embryology
Leiden University
PO Box 9602
2300 RC Leiden
The Netherlands

**P. Jeanty**
Women's Health Care Group
Baptist Hospital
4th Floor, 300, 20th Ave. North
Nashville,
Tennessee 37203
USA

**G. Pilu**
Clinica Ginecologica and Ostetrica e
    Fisiopatologia Prenatale
Università degli Studi di Bologna
Via Massarenti 13
40138 Bologna
Italy

**D. Prandstraller**
Department of Obstetrics and Gynecology
Section of Prenatal Pathophysiology
Bologna University Medical School
Bologna
Italy

**G. Rizzo**
Clinic of Obstetrics and Gynecology
University of Rome 'Tor Vergata'
Policlinico Nuovo S. Eugenio
P. le Umanesimo 10
00144 Rome
Italy

**J. W. Wladimiroff**
University Hospital Rotterdam
Dr Molewaterplein 40
3015 GD Rotterdam
The Netherlands

# Color plates

**Color plate A** Normal four-chamber view at 11 weeks + 3 days of gestation as visualized by transvaginal color-coded Doppler echocardiography. The spine is localized at 7 o'clock. The color-coded Doppler allows discrimination of the inflow into both ventricles

**Color plate B** Short-axis view showing the normal relation of the great arteries at 12 weeks + 2 days. The 'circle and sausage' is visualized with the aortic root in the middle ('circle'). The right ventricular outflow tract lies in front of the aorta and the main pulmonary artery can be seen crossing over the aorta from ventral to dorsal ('sausage' coded in blue)

**Color plates C–G** Hypoplastic left heart at 14 weeks + 3 days of gestation. (C) In the four-chamber view, only one large atrium, one atrioventricular (AV) valve and one large ventricle were visible. (D) In the short-axis view, a large pulmonary trunk (PT) with a bifurcation (marked between the crosses) was visualized. The ascending aorta (marked with two crosses) seemed to be severely hypoplastic; (E) transvaginal color flow Doppler imaging allowed demonstration of a single ventricular inflow only (red) (A = atrium, V = ventricle); (F) during systole, AV regurgitation was demonstrated (blue mosaic) (A = atrium, V = ventricle); (G) stereomicroscopic picture of the fetal heart showing severe hypoplasia of the aorta, the small size of the aortic arch, and the origin of an aberrant right subclavian artery (A. lusoria) from the posterior wall of the aorta near the origin of the left subclavian artery marked by the clamp. The right atrial appendage and the pulmonary trunk are markedly enlarged. The localization of the left ventricle is marked by the marginal branches of the anterior descending coronary artery (on the right side). Reproduced with permission from Gembruch, U., Knöpfle, G., Bald, R. and Hansmann, M. (1993). Early diagnosis of fetal congenital heart disease by transvaginal echocardiography. *Ultrasound Obstet. Gynecol.*, **3**, 310–17

**Color plate H** Color Doppler demonstration of a complete atrioventricular septal defect in a midtrimester fetus

**Color plate I** Cross-section of the upper chest of a third-trimester fetus with hypoplastic left heart with color Doppler demonstration of great vessels. The large pulmonary artery dwarfs the diminutive aortic arch, within which retrograde blood flow is demonstrated

**Color plate J** Pulmonary atresia with intact ventricular septum. The right chambers appear obviously enlarged. Color and pulsed Doppler ultrasound reveal a systolic regurgitant jet directed from the right ventricle to the right atrium

**Color plate K** Parasagittal view of the fetal trunk showing the confluence of the inferior vena cava (IVC), ductus venosus (DV) and hepatic vein (HV) before entering in the right atrium

**Color plate L** Apical four-chamber view of the fetal heart during diastole showing the ventricular filling

**Color plate M** Five-chamber view of the fetal heart during systole showing the left ventricle ejection into aorta

**Color plate N** Short-axis view of the fetal heart during systole showing the right ventricle ejection into the pulmonary artery

**Color plate O** Transverse view of the fetal thorax showing the lung perfusion (left side) and (right side) velocity waveforms from a peripheral pulmonary artery (upper panel) and vein (lower panel) in a normal fetus at 34 weeks of gestation. Note the presence of end-diastolic flow in the artery

*continued on p. xiii*

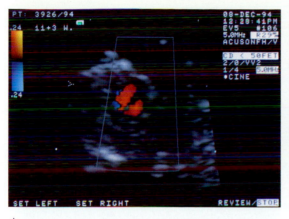

**A**

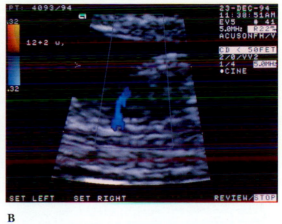

**B**

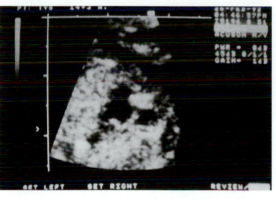

**C**

**D**

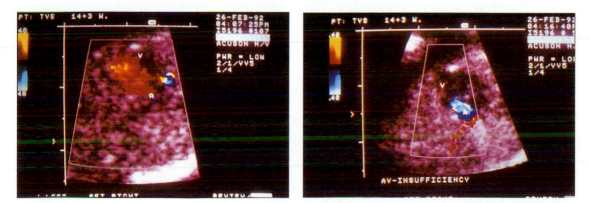

**E**

**F**

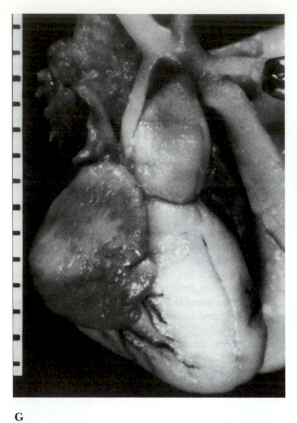

G

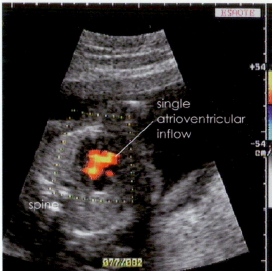

H

single
atrioventricular
inflow

spine

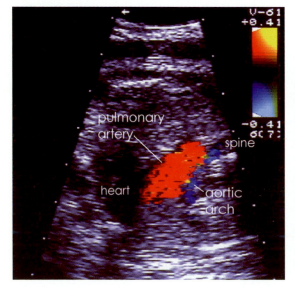

I

pulmonary
artery

spine

heart

aortic
arch

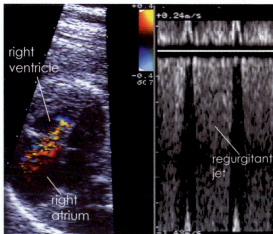

J

right
ventricle

right
atrium

regurgitant
jet

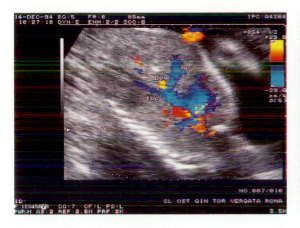

**K**

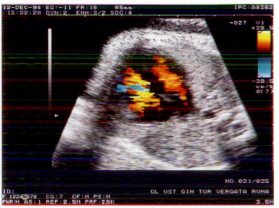

**L**

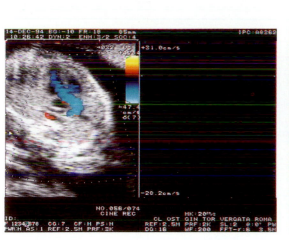

**M**

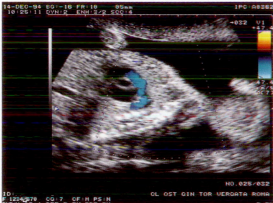

**N**

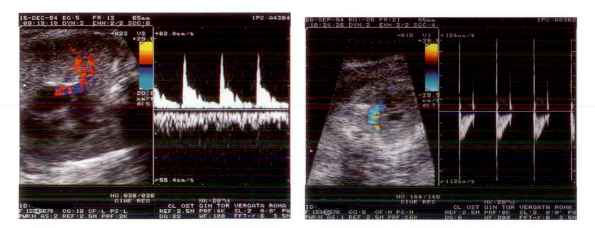

**O**

**P**

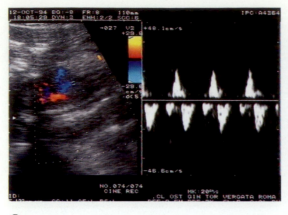

**Q**

**R**

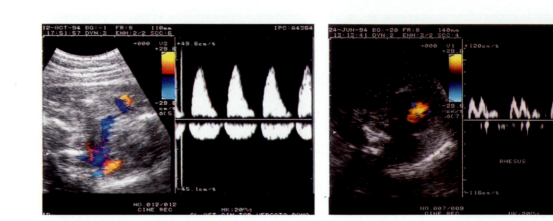

**S**

**T**

**Color plate P** Pulmonary artery velocity waveforms in a severe IUGR fetus at 28 weeks of gestation. The PV is equal to 40 cm/s (normal mean for gestation 62 cm/s) and the TPV 14 ms (normal mean for gestation 34.7 ms)

**Color plate Q** Inferior vena cava velocity waveforms in a severe IUGR fetus at 28 weeks of gestation. The percentage reverse flow is 48.3% (normal mean for gestation 10.5)

**Color plate R** Ductus venosus velocity waveforms in a severe IUGR fetus at 28 weeks of gestation. The flow is reversed during atrial contraction (upper panel)

**Color plate S** Velocity waveforms from umbilical artery (upper panel) and vein (lower panel) in a severe IUGR fetus at 28 weeks of gestation. The end-diastolic flow in umbilical artery is absent and the venous flow shows end-diastolic pulsation

**Color plate T** Velocity waveforms from the tricuspid valve at 28 weeks of gestation in a pregnancy complicated by rhesus isoimmunization 30 min after intravascular transfusion. The E/A is equal to 1

# Foreword

During the last two decades, major new developments in diagnostic ultrasound have revolutionized our knowledge of normal and abnormal fetal cardiac anatomy and function. The introduction of color-coded Doppler facilities has further refined the diagnostic potential of ultrasound in fetal cardiology. Basic knowledge of cardiac development is a prerequisite for a proper interpretation of abnormal sonographic findings. Moreover, insight is needed into the intricate relationship between form and function of the developing heart. The chick embryo model is now providing us with more exciting clues regarding the impact of disturbed neural crest cell migration on cardiac morphology and function.

The prenatal diagnosis and treatment of cardiac rate and rhythm disturbances represent another rapidly expanding area of interest in the field of fetal cardiology. Treatment of supraventricular tachycardia can be considered one of the few truly successful modalities in fetal therapy, particularly in the absence of fetal hydrops.

Data on outcome of congenital heart disease in childhood, as provided by the Baltimore–Washington study, are essential for us to appreciate the clinical significance of prenatal diagnosis of congenital heart disease. There is, however, a note of caution. Whereas specialized centers are instrumental in the enhancement of fetal cardiovascular research, the efficacy of a basic cardiac scan, such as the four-chamber view, is still disappointingly low in a day-to-day obstetric out-patient setting. Here lies a task for all those who are involved in ultrasound training.

The Editors hope that this international undertaking will be helpful to all physicians active in the care of the unborn child.

*Juriy W. Wladimiroff*
*Gianluigi Pilu*

# Normal cardiac development 1

*A. C. Gittenberger-de Groot, M. M. Bartelings, M. C. De Ruiter and R. E. Poelmann*

## INTRODUCTION

During embryonic development, organogenesis starts with the formation of the cardiovascular system. As soon as the simple diffusion of nutrients becomes insufficient because of the increase in size of the embryo, this system has to become functional. Cardiovascular development in the human embryo occurs between 3 and 6 weeks after ovulation (Figure 1). During this period, a heart tube is formed from the mesodermally derived cardiogenic plates. This heart tube loops and develops venous, atrial, ventricular and arterial segments interspaced by transitional zones. The cardiac segments become septated and eventually valve formation takes place at the transitional zones in between.

The most consequential structural changes occur during so-called critical periods in cardiac development. It is in such a period that an organ and its contributing cellular structures are most vulnerable because of active differentiation. Disturbance within such a period will result in more or less serious abnormalities of the heart. Figure 1 clearly indicates the timing of crucial differentiation events in cardiogenesis. There is an overlap of major developmental processes, implying that abnormalities may result from disturbance of more than one process at the same time. Moreover, if one process is deregulated, e.g. ventricular septation, this may result in subsequent abnormalities, e.g. abnormal valve formation.

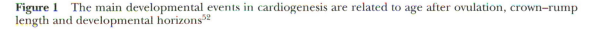

| | | | | | | | | | | | | |
|---|---|---|---|---|---|---|---|---|---|---|---|---|
| HEART TUBE | ------- | | | | | | | | | | | |
| HEART LOOP | ------ | | | | | | | | | | | |
| ATRIAL SEPTATION | | | -------------------------------------------------> | | | | | | | | | |
| VENTRICULAR SEPTATION | | | ------------------------------------ | | | | | | | | |
| CONDUCTION SYSTEM | | | ----------------------------------- | | | | | | | | |
| VALVE FORMATION | | | ------------------------------------------------------> | | | | | | | | | |
| PULMONARY VEINS | | | --------------------- | | | | | | | | | |
| AORTIC ARCH/PULM. ART. | | ------------------------------------ | | | | | | | | | |
| DUCTUS ARTERIOSUS | | | --------------------------------------------> | | | | | | | | | |
| CORONARY VASCULATURE | | | -------------- | | | | | | | | | |
| Ovulation age in days | 18 | 24 | 26 | 28 | 29 | 31 | 33 | 35 | 37 | 39 | 41 | 43 |
| Crown–rump length (mm) | 1.5 | 2-3 | 3.5 | 4-5 | 6-7 | 7-8 | 9-10 | 11-14 | 14-16 | 17-20 | 22-24 | 25-26 |
| Horizons | IX | XI | XII | XIII | XIV | XV | XVI | XVII | XVIII | XIX | XXI | XXII |

**Figure 1** The main developmental events in cardiogenesis are related to age after ovulation, crown–rump length and developmental horizons[52]

Recent advances in molecular biology focusing on the onset and duration of gene expression and their transcription factors in the developing heart allow for a better understanding of both normal and abnormal developmental processes. Basic research in this field is highly dependent on animal models such as transgenic mice in which genes have been knocked out, up-regulated or ectopically expressed. The discovery of gene abnormalities in the human population leads to a better understanding of congenital heart malformation in the setting of syndromes, such as CATCH 22 or in the setting of inheritable muscle diseases such as cardiomyopathies[1,2].

In this chapter, the major events in cardiac development will be discussed and examples of abnormal development, which have their onset in the embryonic period, will be presented.

## CARDIOGENIC PLATE AND EARLY VESSEL FORMATION

At about 13 days after ovulation, the yolk sac (vitelline) and the umbilical extra-embryonic vascular systems develop. They join the intra-embryonic (cardinal) vascular system at about 21 days of development at which the functional state of the circulatory system, including a pumping heart, is reached[3]. The heart, as a specialized part of the cardiovascular system, develops from two cardiogenic plates (Figure 2a) in the splanchnic mesoderm that forms the floor of the celomic cavity. Recent research in animal models reveals that the cardiomyocytes differentiate from cells of the cardiogenic plate. With regard to the origin of the endocardial cells lining the myocardial heart tube on the inside, a dual origin is proposed. One population is supposed to have the same origin as the

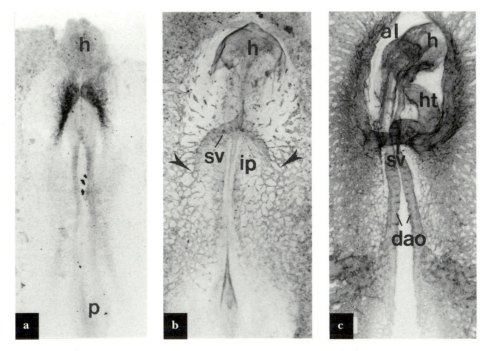

**Figure 2** (a) Dorsal view of a quail embryo (HH 10−) showing the dual origin of the cardiogenic plates, that have not fused in the midline. At this stage the cardiogenic plate stains with a neurofilament antibody RMOL: p, primitive streak; h, head region, 28 ×. (b). Dorsal view of a quail embryo (HH 10) whole mount stained with an anti-endothelial antibody QH1. Endothelial cells are present in the now fused cardiogenic plate area that is already remodeled to form the sinus venosus (sv). In this area there is a connection with the vasculature of the yolk sac (arrows): ip, intestinal portal; h, head region. (c) Dorsal view of a quail embryo (HH 13) stained like the embryo depicted in (b). There is now clearly a sinus venosus (sv), an endocardial heart tube (ht) that connects by way of the first aortic arch arteries (aI) to the dorsal aortae (dao), 24 ×

endothelial cells that line the intra- and extra-embryonic vessels, while a second population is presumed to differentiate from the cardiogenic plate (Figure 2b)[4,5].

Initially, the cardiac celomic cavity has a horseshoe shape, with its bow in the rostral part of the embryo and the open ends at the caudal part. With the formation of the head-fold, the mesoderm of the cardiogenic area is brought from a rostral into a ventral position underneath the head-fold of the embryo. After disappearance of the so-called ventral mesoderm, the developing heart has a dorsal mesocardium connecting a venous pole that is embedded in the mesoderm of the septum transversum and an arterial pole that extends into the splanchnic mesoderm in the pharyngeal arch region (Figure 2c). The septum transversum harbors the developing liver and will contribute to the diaphragm separating thorax and abdomen.

The venous pole of the heart in this area receives blood from both the extra- and the intra-embryonic veins. The arterial end of the heart tube connects by way of the two first aortic arch arteries to the right and left dorsal aortae, which course dorsally along the gut in the splanchnic mesoderm and join the umbilical arteries which run to the placenta.

## HEART TUBE

The endocardial heart tube is formed from an endothelium-lined vessel network which is remodeled to form just a single tube (Figure 2b, c)[5–7]. As described above, a dual origin is suggested for this endocardium. With the invagination of the cardiogenic plates into the celomic (pericardial) cavity, the myocardium or outer wall layer of the heart is formed[8]. The epicardium that will eventually cover the myocardium is extracardiac in origin and develops later. Between the endocardium and the myocardium, a layer of cardiac jelly is formed that is considered to be produced by the myocardial cells[9,10].

The dorsal mesocardium, formed during the invagination, initially connects the heart tube with the dorsal splanchnic mesoderm. Later in development, the major (middle) part of the dorsal mesocardium disappears, leaving the arterial and the venous poles of the heart as the sole connections with the splanchnic mesoderm of the embryonic body[11].

## LOOPING OF THE HEART TUBE

Looping of the heart tube inside the pericardial cavity, with the arterial and the venous poles fixed, is a highly autonomous process[12]. Experiments have shown that this process is largely independent of hemodynamic influences[13]. Generally, the heart tube loops rightward. The mechanism underlying this asymmetric development is still not completely understood. Recent data indicate that this process is under the control of early embryonic regulatory genes[14] and growth factors[15].

During looping, the heart tube develops several sequential segments, separated by more or less distinct boundaries, so-called transitional zones. These show as external grooves and internal reliefs, enabling the following distinction: a sinus venosus segment, a sinu-atrial transition, an atrial segment, an atrioventricular canal, a ventricular inlet segment, a primary fold or bulboventricular transition, a proximal outlet segment, a distal outlet segment which may be considered part of the ventriculo-arterial transition and an aortic sac connecting to the pharyngeal arch arteries (Figure 3). The transitional zones are highly significant for septation, valve formation and the development of the conducting system[11,16].

The formation of the heart loop is completed at the end of the 4th week of development (Figures 4a, b; 5), when most processes concerning the refinement of its inner architecture start (Figure 1).

## ATRIAL SEPTATION AND SINUS VENOSUS INCORPORATION

The sinus venosus, initially part of the vascular system, is incorporated into the posterior wall of the atrial segment (Figure 6b). Recent data on investigation in both chicks and mammals supports earlier studies that the sinus venosus is incorporated not only into the future right

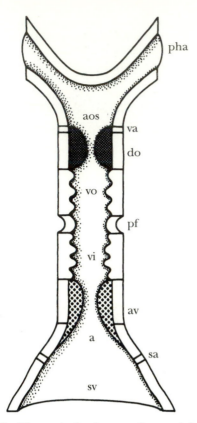

**Figure 3** Theoretical scheme of a straight heart tube showing the sequential segments and transitional zones, going from the venous pole: sv, sinus venosus; sa, sinu-atrial transition; a, atrium; av, atrio-ventricular canal; vi, ventricular inlet; pf, primary fold; vo, proximal ventricular outlet; do, distal outlet; va, ventriculo-arterial transition; and aos, aortic sac to the pharyngeal arch arteries (pha) at the arterial pole

atrium but also into the posterior wall of the left atrium[11,17]. The sinu-atrial transition thus encompasses the pulmonary veins (see separate paragraph) and contributes to the formation of the right and left venous valves. The left venous valve, containing extracardiac mesenchyme, connects to the posterior wall of the aorta and thus to the fibrous heart skeleton[18]. During this process, the left anterior and posterior cardinal veins become obsolete, leaving the coronary sinus as a persisting vessel connecting to the right atrium (Figure 6d).

Atrial septation is a complicated process in which several septa are involved. Between the 4th and the 5th weeks of development the septum primum is completed. Partly overlapping in time, this is followed by the formation of the septum secundum. A complete separation of the left and right atria is not effected in the embryonic and fetal period, however, because the septum primum perforates, forming the ostium secundum (Figure 7). This opening, in combination with the free rim (limbus fossa ovalis) of the septum secundum, forms the foramen ovale. The right venous valve forms the Eustachian and the Thebesian valves, which guard the inferior caval vein and the coronary sinus, respectively. The left venous valve, the septum primum and part of the septum secundum join in the formation of the dorsal part of the atrial septum (Figure 8).

Definitive closure of the atrial septum is only effected after birth, when the valvula foraminis ovalis (septum primum) is pushed against the limbus fossae ovalis (septum secundum) with the increase of the left atrial pressure.

## VENTRICULAR SEPTATION

Ventricular septation takes place between the 4th and 6th weeks of development (Figure 1). It is an intricate process in which several septal components act in concert. Only proper outgrowth and alignment of particular parts will result in a normal ventricular septation. The main parts of the heart tube that are involved are the ventricular inlet and the outlet segment (Figure 6a). In early development, they are separated by a transitional zone called the primary fold, or, in earlier literature, the bulboventricular fold[11]. Recent literature[11,19] shows that the posterior part of the primary fold splits and forms a small gutter that will develop into the right ventricular inlet. This process leads to concurrent formation of the ventricular inlet septum[11] and the trabecular septum. Schematic Figures 6b and 6d depict this process, explaining the expansion of the tricuspid orifice above the inlet of the right ventricle. The posterior wall of the right ventricle is thus a relatively late structure.

In the distal outlet segment lined by endocardial outlet cushions, a septation takes place,

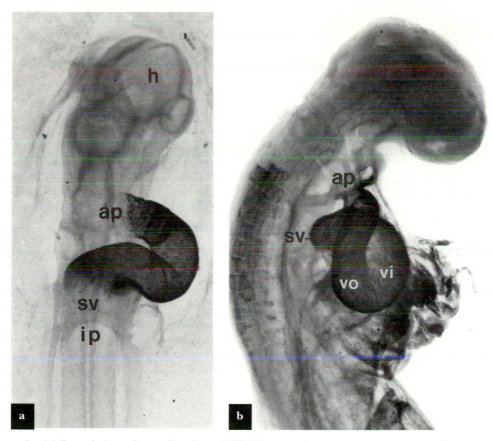

**Figure 4** (a) Dorsal view of a quail embryo (HH 12) stained whole mount for α-actin. The myocardium of the looping heart tube is heavily stained, 40 ×. (b) View from the right side of the looped heart tube of a quail embryo (HH 16) stained as in embryo (a), 34 ×; sv, sinus venosus; ip, intestinal portal; ap, arterial pole; h, head region; vi, ventricular inlet; vo, ventricular outlet

resulting in the formation of a muscular structure which brings the short subaortic part of the initial outlet segment into connection with the left ventricular inlet segment (Figures 6a, c). The main part of the outlet segment contributes to the future right ventricle. Already in the unseptated outflow segment, the arterial orifice level has a saddle shape resulting in a relative lower position of the future aortic orifice (Figures 6a, c). This complicated architecture has as a consequence that, with the septation of the outflow segment, a muscular subpulmonary infundibulum is formed, rather than a true septum. The intercalated valve swelling (the future non-facing or non-coronary semilunar cusp) of the aortic orifice is situated close to the upper endocardial atrioventricular cushion[20,21]. Condensed mesenchyme of the so-called aorto–pulmonary septum subdivides the arterial pole at the orifice level and extends two limbs into the endocardial outlet cushions, which adhere to the myocardium of the outflow segment. Research with chick and mouse models shows that this condensed mesenchyme contains embryonic neural crest cells[22]. The exact function of these cells needs further evaluation. Syndromes in human, e.g. CATCH 22[2], have, as a common denominator, abnormalities in neural crest behavior.

The endocardial cushion tissue, which lines both the atrioventricular canal and a large part of the outlet segment, does not seem to

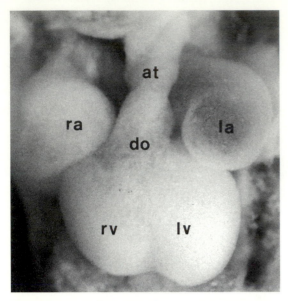

**Figure 5** Ventral view of a human embryonic heart of 5½ weeks gestation. The looping is completed bringing the distal outlet (do) and arterial trunk (at) in between the right atrium (ra) and left atrium (la). The future right (rv) and left (lv) ventricles can already be distinguished. Septation is not yet completed, 13 ×

contribute substantially to the interventricular septum. It is important as a sealing substance, acting as a 'glue' between the various muscular septal components[23]. The last part of the interventricular foramen closes in a 16–17-mm human embryo (Figure 1).

## CONDUCTION SYSTEM

Development of the cardiac conduction system is a provoking subject at the moment. Recent immunohistochemical studies show a protein pattern that explains how the heart can function as a pump before the onset of differentiation of the specialized conducting myocardium[24,25].

The primary heart tube is able to propel the blood forward by peristaltic contraction of the segments, which have alternating slow and fast conduction. In general, it can be said that those segments that are lined by cardiac jelly and that have a smooth myocardium are 'slow' in their

conduction whereas the trabeculated myocardium is 'fast'. Based on classical light microscopic studies, a concept for the development of the specialized cardiac conduction system was based on the presence of four rings of specialized myocardium situated at the transition of the cardiac segments[16]. With the looping of the heart tube, parts of these rings become positioned at the site where the definitive conduction system is formed. It is essential to assume that other parts of the rings disappear during development, e.g. the connection by so-called internodal pathways between the atrial sinus node and the atrioventricular node. The existence of internodal pathways in the fully developed heart has lead to controversy in the literature[26]. Immunohistochemical techniques using an anti-neural crest cell antibody (GIN) have lead to the insight that the primary fold (bulboventricular fold) between the inlet segment and the outlet segment of the embryonic ventricles is important for the development of the atrioventricular part of the conduction system[27]. This primary fold coalesces in the inner curvature of the heart tube with the right side of the atrioventricular canal. This explains the overlap of GIN positivity around the right atrioventricular canal but not around the left (Figures 9a, b) part[11]. There is no evidence that the specialized conduction system derives from the neural crest cells, as has been suggested[28]. Eventually, the heart has an atrial sinus node situated at the anterior basis of the right superior caval vein. This node does not seem to be connected by specific pathways to the atrioventricular node, which is situated in the area of the right atrial septum close to the entrance of the coronary sinus. By way of the bundle of His or the atrioventricular bundle, the fibrous trigone is passed and the top of the interventricular septum is reached. At this site, the bundle divides into a right and a left bundle branch. The development of the fan-like left bundle branch remains an unsolved problem in all current developmental concepts.

In abnormal hearts, immunohistochemistry has shown that the fibers crossing both the left and the right fibrous atrioventricular rings, as seen in the Wolff–Parkinson White syndrome,

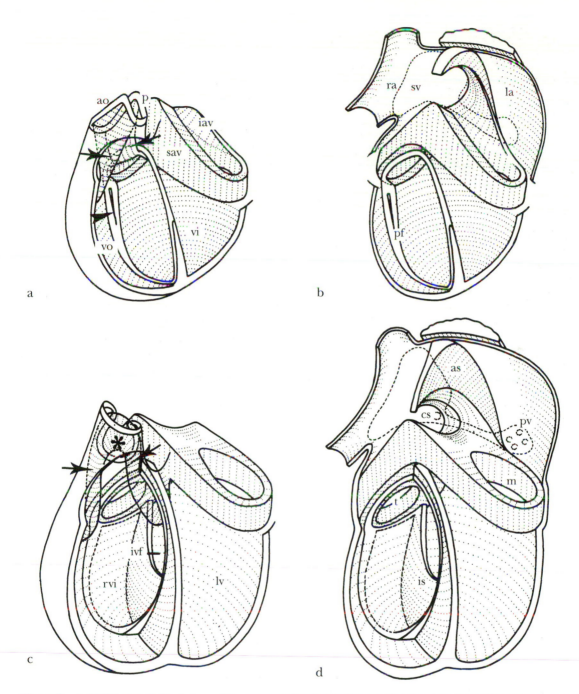

**Figure 6** (a,b) Schematic depiction of the preseptation looped heart tube showing the various segments and transitional zones. (a) Identical drawing as in (b) showing the distal outlet and ventriculo-arterial transition. The atrial and sinus venosus parts have been omitted. In the atrioventricular canal and distal outlet, endocardial cushions are present. These are the superior (sav) and the inferior atrioventricular cushion (iav) and the endocardial outlet ridges (arrows). (c,d) Schematic drawing at the stage of ventricular inlet septation and atrial septation. The right ventricular inlet (rvi) is a newly formed area from a small gutter in the primary fold (arrowhead in (a)). The inlet septum (is) is formed in the same process. (c) Identical drawing as (a) showing an older stage in which the outflow tract ridges are forming an outflow tract septum (asterisk). For abbreviations see also Figure 3. ra, right atrium; as, atrial septum; la, left atrium; m, mitral orifice; t, tricuspid orifice; pv, pulmonary veins; ao, aortic orifice; p, pulmonary orifice; lv, left ventricle; ivf, interventricular foramen

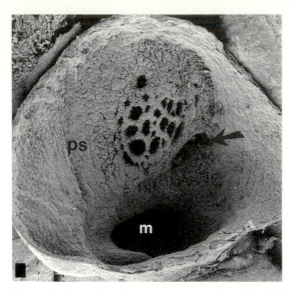

**Figure 7** Scanning electronmicrograph of the left atrium of a HH 25 chick embryo. The perforations in the primary septum (ps) are clear as well as the entrance site of the pulmonary veins (arrow); m, mitral orifice

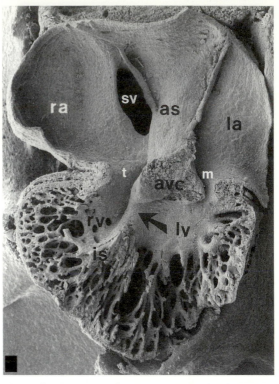

**Figure 8** Scanning electronmicrograph of a HH 28 chick embryo heart, showing the entrance of the sinus venosus (sv) into the right atrium. The dorsal part of the atrial septum (as) is continuous with the atrioventricular cushion (avc); m, mitral orifice; t, tricuspid orifice; ivf, interventricular foramen (arrow); is, inlet septum; rv, right ventricle; lv, left ventricle; ra, right atrium; la, left atrium

consist of working myocardium and are not of conduction system nature.

## ATRIOVENTRICULAR VALVE FORMATION

The opinion, that the superior and the inferior endocardial cushions (Figures 6b, d; 8) are to become the atrioventricular valves, has been commonly held for a long time[29,30]. Other studies have shown that, with the formation of atrioventricular valves, both invagination of the extracardiac mesenchyme and delamination from the underlying myocardium are essential[9,16,18,23]. The endocardial cushions and myocardium that are involved in the formation of the atrioventricular valves are derived from various sources. Between the right atrium and right ventricular inlet, the tricuspid valve is formed, being composed of septal, posterior and anterior leaflets. On the left side, there is the mitral valve with mural and aortic leaflets (Figure 10). Histological differentiation of the atrioventricular cushions into fibrous leaflets is

a relatively late process and the septal leaflet of the tricuspid valve in humans only develops as a separate entity in fetal life.

This implies that abnormal ventricular septation might have consequences for atrioventricular valve formation. Abnormalities in inlet septation, such as atrioventricular septal defects, lead to abnormal atrioventricular valve configurations. Also a deficient expansion of the right part of the atrioventricular canal and inadequate formation of the inlet of the right ventricle can result in abnormalities on a scale ranging from tricuspid atresia to straddling tricuspid valve and double inlet left ventricle.

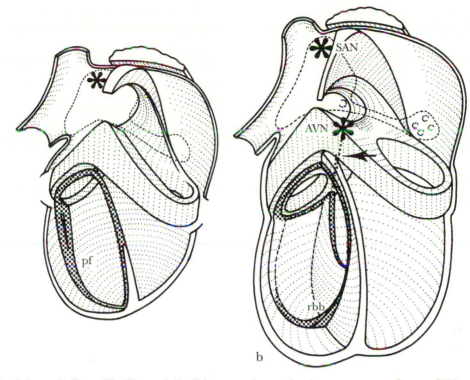

**Figure 9** Schematic figure like Figure 6 (b, d) but now the conduction system according to GIN staining has been indicated in dots. In the early stage (a) the primary fold precedes the formation of the atrioventricular conduction system later on (b). AVN, atrioventricular node; rbb, right bundle branch; left bundle branch not shown (obscured by interventricular septum); atrioventricular bundle, (arrow); SAN, sinu-atrial node

## SEMILUNAR VALVE FORMATION

Semilunar valve formation takes place at the so-called arterial orifice level at the distal end of the ventricular outlet segment. In the early human embryo, this level is saddle-shaped; it is demarcated by the borderline of myocardial tissue (lined on the inside by endocardial outlet ridges) and the mesenchymal tissue, which forms the wall of the aortic sac (Figures 6b, d). After septation at the arterial orifice level by the aorto-pulmonary septum in the 16–17-mm embryo (Figure 1), three semilunar cusps are formed in both the aortic and the pulmonary orifices (Figure 10). The two orifices are already almost in their final position[20]. In each of them, there are two facing cusps, derived from the distal part of the outlet ridges, and one non-facing cusp, derived from the intercalated valve swellings. It is still unclear to what extent invagination of extracardiac mesenchyme is involved

in semilunar cusp formation[31]. Recent data from our own group using retroviral tracing techniques[22] and from literature[32] using chicken–quail chimeras show that neural crest cells are deposited in the semilunar valves. Their actual function is still unknown.

## AORTIC ARCH, PULMONARY ARTERIES AND DUCTUS ARTERIOSUS

Developmentally, the aortic arch, the pulmonary trunk and arteries and the ductus arteriosus are closely related. The description of their embryonic origin in the early part of this century by Congdon[33] has been the basis for further research. The knowledge that there is a remodeling of an initially symmetric system of six (in fact five because the fifth does not develop properly) aortic arch arteries (Figure 11),

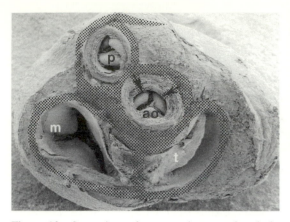

**Figure 10** Scanning electronmicrograph of the base of an embryonic chick heart (HH 34) showing the aortic (ao), pulmonary (p), tricuspid (t) and mitral (m) orifices. The semilunar valves that develop from the endocardial outlet ridges are still thick, like the atrioventricular cushions in the tricuspid and mitral orifices. The sites of coronary endothelial precursors are indicated by a dotted overlay and the ingrowth sites into the aorta by arrows

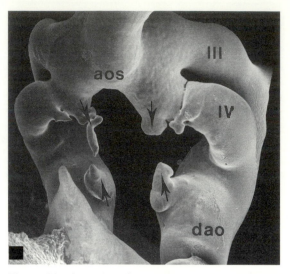

**Figure 11** Scanning electronmicrograph of a cast of the aortic arch arteries in a rat embryo (12 days). The IIIrd and IVth artery are completely developed on both sides. The VIth artery is being formed from a dorsal sprout (arrow) from the dorsal aorta (dao) and a ventral sprout (arrow) from the aortic sac (aos)

combined with migrations and disappearance of various parts, has led to a number of quite satisfactory hypotheses concerning the origin of abnormalities[34].

Recent investigations have led to a re-evaluation of the importance of the early splanchnic vascular system, consisting of isolated endothelial precursors that take part in formation and remodeling of vessels. This system turns out to have a high plasticity[35]. The development of the sixth or pulmonary arch gives rise to the ductus arteriosus which is intricately involved in the formation of the pulmonary arteries[35,36]. It has been shown that the future ductus arteriosus forms the uppermost vessel of a transient system of postbranchial splanchnic arteries which run towards the developing pulmonary region. These connections are already present in a 4–5-mm embryo (Figure 1), while the fourth arch artery is still being formed. As soon as the sixth arch artery becomes functional, the remaining connections between the aorta and the pulmonary region disappear. The origin of the bronchial arteries could be traced as a relatively late system that hooks up to the already present intrapulmonary vascular network[35].

It is hypothesized that these connections may persist, for instance in pulmonary atresia, as so-called major aorto-pulmonary collaterals, which are histologically very similar to the ductus arteriosus[37,38].

Experimental research of neural crest contribution and hemodynamic influences have shown that both have an important part in outflow tract and aortic arch formation[39].

## PULMONARY VEIN FORMATION

This subject deserves special attention as abnormal pulmonary venous development can result in partial to total abnormal venous returns, from (supra)cardial to infracardial (infradiaphragmatic) location[40]. Similar to development of the arterial aortic arch artery system, there is also an initial system of venous drainage by way of splanchnic veins to the right and left superior cardinal veins. Use of the quail embryo and a quail-specific anti-endothelial antibody showed the already formed vessels and the early endothelial precursors and strands. This revealed the connection of the future central pulmonary veins to the sinus venosus segment of the embryonic heart[35] prior to the incorporation of the sinus venosus into the posterior wall of the right and left atrium (Figures 6d; 7)[17]. Restudy of mouse and human embryos showed that this finding might also be relevant in mammals. The implication for abnormal pulmonary venous return, either partial or complete, would be that inadequate incorporation of the sinus venosus could explain most of the abnormalities. This differs from theories that explain abnormal venous connection to the atria by abnormal atrial septation or abnormally positioned outgrowth of pulmonary veins. The supracardial and infracardial connections would reflect persistence of early splanchnic connections to the sinus venosus region and the surrounding large cardiac veins.

## CORONARY VASCULATURE AND EPICARDIUM FORMATION

Until recently, it was generally accepted that the development of the coronary vasculature arose from three sources, namely the endocardium-lined trabeculae of the myocardium; a subepicardial system; and the sprouts of the aortic orifice[41]. It is still an open question whether we are really dealing with three different systems. Recent investigations point towards the subepicardial system being the main source. The heart is covered during development by an epicardial layer that grows out from the celomic wall in the sinus venosus region. A complete covering of the heart tube is established, while the first endothelial precursors move within the subepicardial space and populate the surface of the heart[42]. The main endothelial concentrations are found in the atrioventricular sulcus and at the arterial orifice level, the so-called peritruncal ring (Figure 10). With regard to the development of the origin of the main coronary arteries and the possible aberrations, such as a coronary artery that arises from a pulmonary orifice, it has been demonstrated that aberrant connections can neither be explained by abnormal septation at the arterial orifice level, nor by the initial development of more sprouts from the various semilunar sinuses of both the aortic and the pulmonary orifices[43]. Septation takes place well before the development of the coronary orifices at about 16–17-mm (Figure 1). In an extensive study concerning human, rat and mouse hearts, only two coronary arterial ostia were seen. These always developed in the facing semilunar sinuses of the aortic orifice. These main coronary arterial connections and ostia are formed by a penetrating ingrowth mechanism. This ingrowth has been confirmed by quail–chicken chimera experiments, showing both intramyocardial and main stem coronary origin from the implanted quail cells[44]. The differentiation into a venous and an arterial coronary vasculature takes place at a somewhat later stage. The veins drain either into the coronary sinus, or as individual branches into the right atrium of the heart.

## CARDIAC EMBRYONIC MALDEVELOPMENT

Detailed knowledge of cardiac embryology enables an insight into the various stages of cardiac development in which congenital abnormalities might find their origin. Evidently, the period between the 3rd and the 8th week of development is important. More insight is needed into the cardiac genes that are expressed during this period. A detailed insight with regard to the exact sequence and timing of the developmental events may allow the disproving of certain theories, such as some of those explaining the aberrant origin of coronary arteries from the pulmonary orifice, e.g. by abnormal septation[43,44].

It should be emphasized that different developmental routes may eventually result in (nearly) identical abnormalities in the neonatal period, which may present themselves as a single entity. This principle is exemplified by cases of persistent ductus arteriosus that seem identical in clinical behavior. Careful histological studies have revealed that we are in fact dealing with a mixture of different forms[45]. The most common type of persistent ducti is a congenital malformation with an unknown etiology. Maybe it has a genetic background, as has been described for the dog[46]. These ducti clearly differ in histology from cases of persistent ductus arteriosus induced by rubella infection[47].

A second example can be provided from our experimental embryonic studies that were designed to differentiate between hemodynamic and direct neural crest disturbances in the understanding of outflow tract malformations of the heart. Especially double outlet right ventricle can be evoked by a variety of causes such as neural crest ablation[48], all-*trans* retinoic acid application[49,50] and rerouting of the venous blood flow[39]. Transgenic mice with either ectopic expression of genes or knock-out phenotypes share comparable cardiovascular abnormalities.

Relevant for early fetal diagnosis of abnormalities by echocardiography are those malformations that persist or become even more pronounced during cardiac histogenesis in the months following the embryonic period. In the histogenesis phase, there can be an increase of, for example, stenosis or hypoplasia, even up to the stage of atresia. Secondary pathology, such as endocardial fibroelastosis and calcification can also develop. There are also indications that abnormalities such as small muscular ventricular septal defects can disappear.

Two cardiac structures are exceptional in that they complete their development only after birth. These are the patent foramen ovale and the patent ductus arteriosus[51]. Prenatal closure can lead to intrauterine fetal distress or even death.

For adequate intrauterine diagnosis, it is essential to expand research into both the embryonic and fetal stages of cardiovascular development. Increase of our knowledge into regulation of genes will allow a better understanding of the morphogenetic processes that underlie abnormal development. Future goals may be directed towards prevention and intrauterine therapy of cardiac abnormalities.

# References

1. Fananapazir, L. and Epstein, N. D. (1994). Genotype–phenotype correlations in hypertrophic cardiomyopathy: insights provided by comparisons of kindreds with distinct and identical β-myosin heavy chain gene mutations. *Circulation*, **89**, 22–32
2. Wilson, D. I., Burn, J., Scrambler, P. and Goodship, J. (1993). DiGeorge syndrome: part of CATCH 22. *J. Med. Genet.*, **30**, 852–6
3. Arey, L. B. (1966). The primitive vascular system. *Developmental Anatomy. A Textbook and Laboratory Manual of Embryology*, pp. 347–9. (Philadelphia, London: W. B. Saunders)
4. Eisenberg, L. M. and Markwald, R. R. (1995). Molecular regulation of atrioventricular valvuloseptal morphogenesis. *Circ. Res.*, **77**, 1–6
5. Gittenberger-de Groot, A. C., De Ruiter, M. C. and Poelmann, R. E. (1996). Vasculogenesis and vessel wall differentiation in the embryo. *Basic and Applied Myology*, **6**, 5–12
6. Patten, B. M. (1968). The development of the heart. In Gould, S. E. (ed.) *Pathology of the Heart and Blood Vessels*, 3rd edn. pp. 20–90. (Springfield, Illinois: Charles C. Thomas)
7. Coffin, D. J. and Poole, T. J. (1988). Embryonic vascular development: immunohistochemical identification of the origin and subsequent morphogenesis of the major vessel primordia in quail embryos. *Development*, **102**, 735–48
8. DeRuiter, M. C., Poelmann, R. E., VanderPlas-de Vries, I., Mentink, M. M. T. and Gittenberger-de Groot, A. C. (1992). The development of the myocardium and endocardium in mouse embryos. Fusion of two heart tubes? *Anat. Embryol.*, **185**, 461–73
9. Manasek, F. J. (1975). The extracellular matrix of the early embryonic heart. In Lieberman, M. and Sano, T. (eds.) *Developmental and Physiological Correlates of Cardiac Muscle*, pp. 1–20. (New York: Raven Press)
10. Wunsch, A. M., Little, C. D. and Markwald, R. R. (1994). Cardiac endothelial heterogeneity defines valvular development as demonstrated by the diverse expression of JB3, an antigen of the endocardial cushion tissue. *Dev. Biol.*, **165**, 585–601
11. Gittenberger-de Groot, A. C., Bartelings, M. M. and Poelmann, R. E. (1995). Overview: cardiac morphogenesis. In Clark, E. B., Markwald, R. R. and Takao, A. (eds.) *Developmental Mechanisms of Heart Disease. Proceedings of the Fourth International Symposium on Etiology and Morphogenesis of Congenital Heart Disease*, Chapter 15, pp. 157–68. (Mount Kisco, NY: Futura Press)

12. Nakamura, A., Kulikowski, R. R., Lacktis, J. W. and Manasek, F. J. (1980). Heartlooping: a regulated response to deforming forces. In Van Praagh, R. and Takao, A. (eds.) *Etiology and Morphogenesis of Congenital Heart Disease*, pp. 81–98. (New York: Futura)

13. Manasek, F. J. and Monroe, R. G. (1972). Early cardiac morphogenesis is independent of function. *Dev. Biol.*, **27**, 584–8

14. Wolpert, L. and Brown, N. A. (1995). Hedgehog keeps to the left. *Nature*, **377**, 103–4

15. Yost, H. J. (1990) Inhibition of proteoglycan synthesis eliminates left–right asymmetry in *Xenopus laevis* cardiac looping. *Development*, **110**, 865–7

16. Wenink, A. C. G. (1987). Embryology of the heart. In Anderson, R. H., Macartney, F. J., Shinebourne, E. A. and Tynan, M. (eds.) *Paediatric Cardiology*, Vol. I. pp. 83–107. (Edinburgh, London, Melbourne, New York: Churchill Livingstone)

17. DeRuiter, M. C., Gittenberger-de Groot, A. C., Wenink, A. C. G., Poelmann, R. E. and Mentink, M. M. T. (1995). In normal development pulmonary veins are connected to the sinus venosus segment in the left atrium. *Anat. Rec.*, **243**, 84–92

18. Van Gils, F. A. W. (1981). The fibrous skeleton in the human heart: embryological and pathogenetic considerations. *Virchows Archiv. A. Path. Anat. and Hist.*, **393**, 61–73

19. Wenink, A. C. G., Wisse, L. J. and Groenendijk, P. M. (1994). Development of the inlet portion of the right ventricle in the embryonic rat heart: the basis for tricuspid valve development. *Anat. Rec.*, **239**, 216–23

20. Bartelings, M. M. and Gittenberger-de Groot, A. C. (1988). The arterial orifice level in the human embryo. *Anat. Embryol.*, **177**, 537–42

21. Bartelings, M. M. and Gittenberger-de Groot, A. C. (1988). The outflow tract of the heart – embryologic and morphologic correlations. *Int. J. Cardiol.*, **22**, 289–300

22. Noden, D. M., Poelmann, R. E. and Gittenberger-de Groot, A. C. (1995). Cell origins and tissue boundaries during outflow tract development. *Trends Cardiovas. Med.*, **5**, 69–75

23. Wenink, A. C. G. and Gittenberger-de Groot, A. C. (1985). The role of the atrioventricular cushions in septation of the heart. *Int. J. Cardiol.*, **8**, 25–44

24. Wessels, A., Vermeulen, J. L. M., Virágh, S., Kálmán, F., Lamers, W. H. and Moorman, A. F. M. (1991). Spatial distribution of 'tissue specific' antigens in the developing human heart and skeletal muscle. II. An immunohistochemical analysis of myosin heavychain isoform expression patterns in the embryonic heart. *Anat. Rec.*, **229**, 355–68

25. Moorman, A. F. M. and Lamers, W. H. (1994). Molecular anatomy of the developing heart. *Trends Cardiovasc. Med.*, **4** (6), 257–63

26. Janse, M. J. and Anderson, R. H. (1974). Specialized internodal atrial pathways – fact or fiction? *Eur. J. Cardiol.*, **2-2**, 117–36

27. Wessels, A., Vermeulen, J. L. M. and Verbeek, F. J. (1992). Spatial distribution of tissue-specific antigens in the developing human heart and skeletal muscle: III. An immunohistochemical analysis of the distribution of the neural tissue antigen GLN2 in the embryonic heart; implications for the development of the atrioventricular conduction system. *Anat. Embryol.*, **232**, 97–111

28. Gorza, L., Schiaffino, S. and Vitadello, M. (1988). Heart conduction system: a neural crest derivative? *Brain Res.*, **457**, 360–6

29. Odgers, P. N. B. (1939). The development of the atrioventricular valves in man. *J. Anat.*, **73**, 643–57

30. Ugarte, M., Enriquez de Salamanca, F. and Quero, M. (1976). Endocardial cushion defects. An anatomical study of 54 specimens. *Br. Heart J.*, **38**, 674–82

31. Gittenberger-de Groot, A. C., Bartelings, M. M. and Wenink, A. C. G. (1986). Developmental considerations with regard to normal and abnormal arterial valve formation. In Arntzenius, A. C., Dunning, A. J. and Snellen, H. A. (eds.) *4th Einthoven Meeting on Past and Present Cardiology. Theme: Valvular Disease*, pp. 29–34. (Assen/Maastricht, Wolfeboro, New Hampshire: Van Gorcum)

32. Sunaida, H., Akimoto, N. and Akamura, H. (1989). Distribution of the neural crest cells in the heart of birds: a three-dimensional analysis. *Anat. Embryol.*, **180**, 29–35

33. Congdon, E. D. (1922). Transformation of the aortic-arch system during the development of the human embryo. *Contr. Embryol. Carneg. Inst.*, **14**, 47–110

34. Barry, A. (1951). The aortic arch derivatives in the human adult. *Anat. Rec.*, **111**, 221–38

35. DeRuiter, M. C., Gittenberger-de Groot, A. C., Poelmann, R. E., VanIperen, L. and Mentink, M. M. T. (1993). Development of the pharyngeal arch system related to the pulmonary and bronchial vessels in the avian embryo. With a concept on systemic-pulmonary collateral artery formation. *Circulation*, **87** (4), 1306–19

36. DeRuiter, M. C., Gittenberger-de Groot, A. C., Rammos, S. and Poelmann, R. E. (1989). The special status of the pulmonary arch artery in the branchial system of the rat. *Anat. Embryol.*, **179**, 319–25

37. Haworth, S. G. and Macartney, F. J. (1980). Growth and development of pulmonary circulation in pulmonary atresia with ventricular septal defect and major aorto-pulmonary collateral arteries. *Br. Heart J.*, **44**, 14–24

38. DeRuiter, M. C., Gittenberger-de Groot, A. C., Bogers, A. J. J. C. and Elzenga, N. J. (1994). The restricted surgical relevance of morphologic criteria to classify systemic-pulmonary collateral arteries in pulmonary atresia with ventricular septal defect. *J. Thorac. Cardiovasc. Surg.*, **108**, 692–8

39. Gittenberger-de Groot, A. C., Bartelings, M. M. and Poelmann, R. E. (1995). Normal and abnormal morphogenesis of the outflow tract. In Clark, E. B., Markwald, R. R. and Takao, A. (eds.) *Developmental Mechanisms of Heart Disease. Proceedings of the Fourth International Symposium on Etiology and Morphogenesis of Congenital Heart Disease*, Chapter 25, pp. 249–54. (Mount Kisco, NY: Futura Press)

40. Rammos, S., Gittenberger-de Groot, A. C. and Oppenheimer-Dekker, A. (1990). The abnormal pulmonary venous connection: a developmental approach. *Int. J. Cardiol.*, **29**, 285–95

41. Viragh, S. and Challice, C. E. (1981). The origin of the epicardium and the embryonic myocardial circulation in the mouse. *Anat. Rec.*, **201**, 157–68

42. Vrancken Peeters, M. P. F. M., Mentink, M. M. T., Poelmann, R. E. and Gittenberger-de Groot, A. C. (1995). Cytokeratins as a marker for epicardial development. *Anat. Embr.*, **191**, 503–8

43. Bogers, A. J. J. C., Gittenberger-de Groot, A. C., Dubbeldam, J. A. and Huysmans, H. A. (1988). Inadequacy of the present theories on proximal coronary artery development. *Int. J. Cardiol.*, **20**, 117–23

44. Poelmann, R. E., Gittenberger-de Groot, A. C., Mentink, M. M. T., Bökenkamp, R. and Hogers, B. (1993). Development of the cardiac coronary vascular endothelium, studied with antiendothelial antibodies, in chicken–quail chimeras. *Circ. Res.*, **73**, 559–68

45. Gittenberger-de Groot, A. C. (1977). Persistent ductus arteriosus: most probably a primary congenital malformation. *Br. Heart J.*, **39**, 610–18

46. Gittenberger-de Groot, A. C., Strengers, J. L. M., Mentink, M. M. T., Poelmann, R. E. and Patterson, D. F. (1985). Histologic studies on normal and persistent ductus arteriosus in the dog. *J. Am. Coll. Cardiol.*, **6**, 394–404

47. Gittenberger-de Groot, A. C., Moulaert, A. J. M. and Hitchcock, J. F. (1980). Histology of the persistent ductus arteriosus in cases of congenital rubella. *Circulation*, **62**, 183–6

48. Kirby, M. L. (1989). Plasticity and predetermination of mesencephalic and trunk neural crest transplanted into the region of the cardiac neural crest. *Dev. Biol.*, **134**, 402–12

49. Broekhuizen, M. L. A., Bouman, H. G. A., Mast, F., Mulder, P. G. H., Gittenberger-de Groot, A. C. and Wladimiroff, J. W. (1995). Hemodynamic changes in HH stage 34 chick embryos after treatment with all-trans-retinoic acid. *Pediatr. Res.*, **38** (3), 342–8

50. Pexieder, T., Pfizenmaier Rousseil, M. and Prados-Frutos, J. C. (1992). Prenatal pathogenesis of the transposition of great arteries. In Vogel, M. and Bühlmeyer, K. (eds.), *Transposition of the Great Arteries: 25 years after Rashkind Balloon Septostomy*, pp. 11–27. (Darmstadt: Steinkopff Verlag)

51. Gittenberger-de Groot, A. C., Van Ertbruggen, I., Moulaert, A. J. M. and Harinck, E. (1980). The ductus arteriosus in the preterm infant: histologic and clinical observations. *J. Pediatr.*, **96**, 88–93

52. Sissman, N. J. (1970). Developmental landmarks in cardiac morphogenesis: comparative chronology. *Am. J. Cardiol.*, **25**, 141–8

# A practical approach to the ultrasound investigation of the fetal heart

*P. Jeanty*

2

## INTRODUCTION

Pioneer studies on the ultrasound investigation of the fetal heart were reported in the early 1970s. Since high-resolution real-time ultrasound was introduced in the late 1970s, reports on ultrasound assessment of fetal cardiac anatomy and function have been appearing with increasing frequency both in the obstetric and cardiologic literature. Fetal echocardiography is now a well-established technique for prenatal diagnosis of cardiac heart defects. The diffusion of this technique is limited at present. However, cardiac defects are one of the most common types of congenital anomalies, and we anticipate that routine sonography in the future will include a basic echocardiographic examination. It is clear that this will demand a significant improvement over the present level of expertise and training. The purpose of this chapter is to provide a practical approach to the ultrasound investigation of the fetal heart.

Fetal echocardiography is mostly based upon real-time investigation. We will first describe the normal anatomy in the different planes, then we will review the sequential approach to the heart as it is adapted to the examination of the fetus. Finally, we will consider the use of M-mode and Doppler ultrasound.

## A CHEAP CARDIAC MODEL

The three-dimensional anatomy of the heart is difficult to remember, and it helps to have access to a model of cardiac anatomy. This can easily be achieved using both hands to represent the two ventricles: the left hand represents the left ventricle and the right hand the right ventricle. Hold the left hand with the fourth and fifth digits flexed, while the other digits are moderately extended. Turn the palm so that it faces your chest: this is the left ventricle. The index and third fingers represent the outflow tract and the ascending aorta, the thumb represents the direction of the flow through the mitral valve, and the left wrist is the cardiac apex. Now hold the left hand with the right hand by placing the palm of the right hand over the back of the left hand. The right thumb should be under the left medius, close to the chest. It represents the direction of the flow through the tricuspid valve; the encircling palm represents the right ventricle wrapped around the base of the left ventricle. The right index is the main pulmonary artery. Note that the right index originates to the right and anteriorly to the left index finger. This is the normal relationship of the pulmonary artery to the aorta. Although the exact relationships are not observed, this is a reasonable approximation. Dextrocardia can be similarly reproduced by doing the symmetrical movements of the contralateral hands.

## THE FETAL CIRCULATION

The fetal circulation differs from the adult circulation in many respects. The adult circulation is a *sequential* circulation. If one could travel on a red blood cell, the journey would pass through the right atrium, right ventricle,

15

pulmonary artery, lungs, pulmonary veins, left atrium, left ventricle, aorta and finally back through the cava. Each location is visited sequentially.

In the fetus the situation is different. Let us first travel on a red blood cell that has just returned from the placenta for oxygenation. The journey starts with the umbilical vein, ductus venosus, inferior vena cava and right atrium. Here is the first change: instead of continuing into the right ventricle, the red blood cell will probably go through the foramen ovale into the left atrium, left ventricle, aorta, brachiocephalic vessels, head or upper limbs, then return by the superior vena cava into the right atrium. The blood flow is thus separated in the right atrium into a right heart flow (essentially deoxygenated blood from the head and upper limbs) and a left heart flow (oxygenated blood from the placenta). This results from streaming of the blood as it enters the right atrium.

The eustachian valve (the junctional fold between the inferior vena cava and the right atrium) directs the inferior vena caval flow toward the foramen ovale which is very close to the inferior vena cava. The inferior caval flow itself is divided into two components: the oxygenated blood coming from the left hepatic vein (and ductus) and the desaturated blood from the rest of the inferior vena cava. The oxygenated blood enters the foramen ovale, while the desaturated blood goes through the tricuspid valve[1]. The foramen ovale is bordered on its inferior edge by the septum primum which is in the left atrium. The septum secundum makes the superior border and is on the right atrial side. The foramen ovale opening, thus, is patent for a flow that is oriented from bottom to top and is against the direction of the flow of the superior vena cava which is in the direction of the tricuspid valve. After travelling through the upper part of the body, the red blood cell has lost some of its oxygen and will go on to perfuse the body and obtain a refill in the placenta.

Coming from the superior vena cava, it will go through the tricuspid valve to the right ventricle and pulmonary artery. Here is another change: instead of going through the lungs it will go through a fetal bypass called the *ductus* and arrive directly into the descending aorta. Since the lungs are not ventilated *in utero*, blood would not become oxygenated by passing through them, and only about 10% of the pulmonary circulation perfuses the lungs.

Of course, the separation of the inferior and superior vena cava flows is not perfect, and there is some mixing of the two circulations. Yet, because of the streaming, the most oxygenated blood perfuses the heart and the brain. The fetal circulation is therefore not a sequential circulation, but a *parallel* circulation with a bifurcation at the right atrium into the left or right heart and a bypass at the ductus arteriosus, skipping the left heart.

Another feature of the fetal circulation is the ductus venosus. The ductus venosus allows blood to bypass the hepatic circulation and thus prevent a loss of pressure in the returning circulation. In the lamb, only 40–50% of the flow passes through the hepatic sinusoid, the rest passes through the ductus. This explains why the ductus venosus is difficult to image: if most of the flow passed through the ductus, its caliber would be equal to that of the umbilical vein, which it is not. The ductus venosus is believed to regulate the flow to the fetal heart by preventing overload when uterine contractions express blood from the placenta into the fetal circulation. Although the ductus walls contain smooth muscle, the presence of a sphincter is debated. While some authors have found evidence of a sphincter[2], others have not[3].

In fetal anemia, increased liver hematopoiesis is probably responsible for compression of the venous system which produced the ascites which is observed. In hypoxemic states ('placental insufficiency' for instance) the flow is redistributed so that a constant supply of oxygen is provided to the brain, myocardium and adrenal glands. Blood flow to the lungs decreases progressively, while flow to the gastrointestinal tract, musculoskeletal system and kidneys decreases abruptly[4]. The decreased perfusion of the kidney leads to a decrease in glomerular filtration and production of urine and thus to oligohydramnios.

## REAL-TIME EXAMINATION

The heart can be observed in an infinity of planes, but a few sections form the basis on which most of the diagnoses are made[5]. These planes include the four-chamber, short-axis (or axial), left and right chambers and great vessels views. Although it is convenient to refer to these standardized views for description purposes, in practice it may be difficult to reproduce these exact sections, and the operator should be familiar with small variations of these planes. It is important to examine the heart with the least number of active focal zones on the transducer. This increases the frame rate, decreases blurring due to averaging of systolic and diastolic frames, permits a better motion analysis and allows a true determination of the fetal heart rate. You can easily verify that, when all the focal zones are turned on, the heart rate slows down noticeably, giving a false impression of bradycardia.

### Four-chamber view

The four-chamber view (Figure 1) is obtained by making a section that is practically axial to the fetal chest[6]. The four-chamber view can be obtained either with the long axis of the heart in the axis of the beam or perpendicular to the beam. The orthogonal view is best to study the septum (both interatrial and interventricular) (Figure 2). Otherwise, the sound waves are reflected at a shallow angle and away from the transducer. This creates the appearance of a septal defect.

This section is now part of the routine (Level I) examination and detects roughly one-third of the cardiac anomalies[7]. The important landmarks to identify are the apex of the heart, the base, the interventricular septum, the interatrial septum, the two atrioventricular valves (tricuspid and mitral valve) and the four cavities delineated by these structures. The thicknesses of the interventricular septum and of the free ventricular walls are the same. Notice that the heart is not midline but shifted to the left side of the chest. The axis of the interventricular septum is about 45° to 20° to the left of the anteroposterior axis of the fetus[8]. Because of the

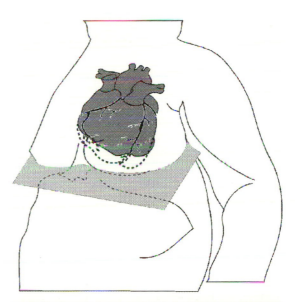

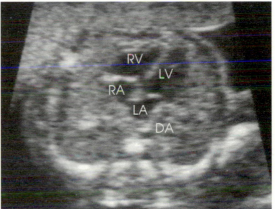

**Figure 1** Upper panel, the four-chamber view of the fetal heart is obtained by a cross-section of the chest. Lower panel, sonographic demonstration of the four-chamber view in a midtrimester fetus. LA, RA, left and right atrium; LV, RV, left and right ventricle; DA, descending aorta

left-sided position of the heart, the right ventricle is anterior and closest to the anterior chest wall, while the left atrium is the most posterior chamber and closest to the spine. These relations are not true in congenital malformations, as we shall see later, but, for now, are convenient simplifications.

Other important landmarks should be recognized. In the right atrium, two thin lines distinct from the interatrial septum can occasionally be seen. The *eustachian valve*, a crest between the

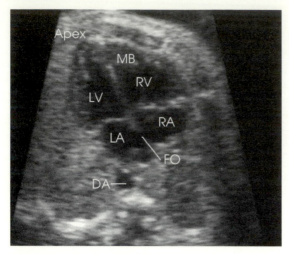

**Figure 2** An orthogonal view of the four cardiac chambers demonstrates the interventricular septum between the left and right ventricles (LV, RV). The interatrial septum is interrupted centrally by the foramen ovalis (FO). The moderator band (MB) is seen at the apex of the right ventricle. Other abbreviations as in previous figures

inferior vena cava and the wall of the right atrium, is located close to the inferior vena cava. The *Chiari network* is composed of abnormal lace-like strands that attach to the eustachian valve and the crista terminalis. It results from the incomplete resorption of the septum spurium which should be completed by the 3rd month and exists in about 1% of patients[9]. The interatrial septum is open at the level of the *foramen ovale*. The foramen ovale flap is visible in the left atrium, beating toward the left side. The insertion of the tricuspid valve along the interventricular septum is more apical than the insertion of the mitral valve. The confluence of the pulmonary veins into the left atrium serves to identify it as such. The most anterior vein is the inferior pulmonary vein; the most posterior is the superior pulmonary vein. The right ventricle appears foreshortened compared to the left because of a large muscle bundle at its apex: the *moderator band*. In favorable cases, one can note the difference in lining of the two ventricles: the right ventricle has a coarser lining than the left due to a coarser trabeculation. Even more difficult to observe is that a papillary muscle (the muscle of the septal leaflet of the tricuspid valve)

implants on the septum in the right ventricle, while the left side of the interventricular septum is free of papillary muscle. In the four-chamber view, both ventricles should have almost the same width (right over left = 1.1).

By turning the transducer while keeping the left ventricle and the aorta in the same plane, one can obtain the left heart views, while the right heart views are obtained by moving the transducer craniad and tilting slightly in the direction of the left shoulder.

## The left heart views

This section (Figure 3) demonstrates important landmarks: the mitral valve is seen between the left atrium and the left ventricle. Note that the posterior leaflet is shorter than the anterior leaflet. The anterior leaflet is in continuity with the posterior wall of the aorta. The anterior wall of the aorta is in continuity with the interventricular septum. The aortic valve can be seen at the base of the aorta.

## The right heart view

This section (Figure 4) demonstrates the right ventricle and the ventricular outflow tract. The main pulmonary artery originates from the anterior ventricle and trifurcates into a large vessel, the ductus going into the descending aorta, and two small vessels, the pulmonary arteries. The pulmonary valve is anterior and cranial to the aortic valve.

## Short-axis view

The appearance of the short-axis view depends on the level at which it is obtained in the heart from the apex to the base. At the apex, a figure *8* is seen with the two ventricles separated by the interventricular septum. Both ventricles have the same morphology and size. Round structures in the ventricular cavities represent sections of papillary muscle. When the section is closer to the base, the valves are visible. The section of the mitral valve has a typical fish-mouth or oval shape; the tricuspid section resembles more an arrowhead. At the base of the

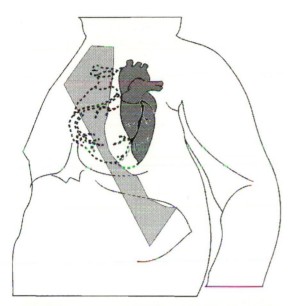

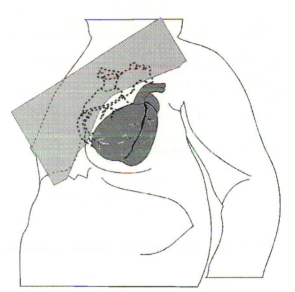

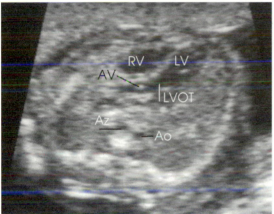

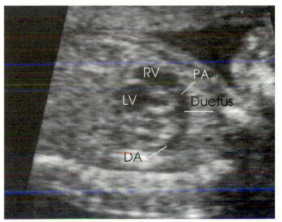

**Figure 3** Upper panel, a view of the left heart is obtained by an oblique section of the fetal chest. Lower panel, long-axis view of the left ventricle (LV) demonstrating the continuity between the outflow tract (LVOT) and the ascending aorta. The aortic valve (AV) is seen. Ao, descending aorta; Az, azygos vein

**Figure 4** Upper panel, a view of the right heart is obtained by an oblique section of the fetal chest. Lower panel, the outflow tract of the right ventricle (RV) is in continuity with the pulmonary artery (PA), within which the pulmonary valve can be seen. The pulmonary artery is seen continuing into the ductus arteriosus which is in turn connected to the descending aorta (DA)

heart, the axial section demonstrates the right heart wrapped around the aorta (Figure 5). The section resembles the Yellow Pages logo ('Let your fingers do the walking'). This section is perpendicular to the ascending aorta and demonstrates the right atrium, tricuspid valve, right ventricle, pulmonary valve, main pulmonary artery and ductus. This is the best section to demonstrate the pulmonary valve.

## The valves

The implantation of the tricuspid valve on the septum is more apical than that of the mitral valve. The tricuspid valve has three leaflets: a large anterior leaflet, a scalloped posterior leaflet and a small septal leaflet. The anterior leaflet of the mitral valve should be in continuity with the posterior wall of the aorta. The anterior leaflet is longer than the posterior leaflet which

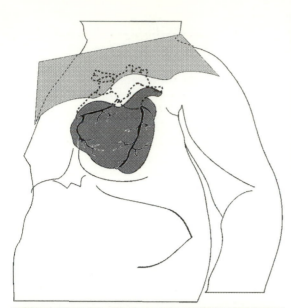

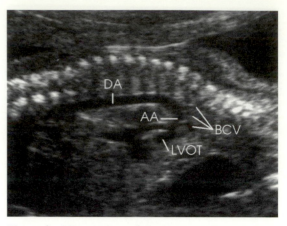

**Figure 6** The aortic arch (AA) is seen giving rise to the brachio-cephalic vessels (BCV). LVOT, outflow tract of left ventricle; DA, descending aorta

## The vessels

There are two *arches* in the fetus and they should be distinguished. The aortic arch (Figure 6) is recognized from the curve of the ductus by the following criteria. The brachiocephalic vessels originate from the aortic arch, while no vessels emanate from the ductus (Figure 4). The curve of the aortic arch is gentler than that of the ductus, which is slightly more angular. The cavae can be seen in a longitudinal view as they both enter the right atrium.

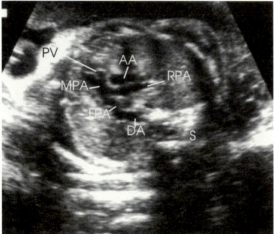

**Figure 5** Upper panel, a short-axis view of the great vessels is obtained by a cross-section of the upper fetal chest. Lower panel, the main pulmonary artery (MPA) surrounds the ascending aorta (AA) thus attesting a normal relationship between the great arteries. The trifurcation of the main pulmonary artery into the left and right pulmonary arteries (LPA, RPA) and the ductus arteriosus (DA) is seen in the same plane. PV, pulmonary valves; S, spine

may be difficult to see. In the short-axis view of the heart, the valves can be seen to make a smaller inner structure within the ventricle. The image of the aortic valve in the short axis of the aorta is an inverted *Y* or *Mercedes-Benz* sign. Sometimes the coronary arteries are visible alongside the aorta.

## Cardiac measurements

Cardiac measurements are simple to obtain and were an easy source of publication in the early days of fetal echocardiography. Some authors have advocated simple measurements that do not require knowledge of the cardiac cycle[10], while others insisted on rigorous frame-by-frame analysis or M-mode tracing to distinguish between the two[11]. Although some authors considered the measurements reliable[12], usually the errors on the measurements are so great that the resulting nomograms are limited to linear regressions. Nomograms of small structures show 5th and 95th confidence limits that encompass variations of size in the 30–80% range[13]; thus, normal variations are greater than the variations induced by pathology. Intraobserver variation can be as great as 40%[14], yet intraobserver variability is usually much smaller than inter-observer variability. The landmarks used for standardization may be altered in malformed hearts, and, finally, most anomalies are easily detectable without using any nomogram. Thus, over the years we have matured to realize that nomograms were not necessary to the diagnosis of cardiac anomalies, and have abandoned even our own cardiac nomograms.

Though measurements are of little help, using other cardiac structures for reference can be quite beneficial, and it is sufficient to keep a few simple rules in mind. The normal heart occupies roughly one-third of the chest. Since the pressure on both sides of the heart is the same (equalized by the ductus and foramen ovale), the workloads are the same too. Thus the heterolateral structures should have similar diameters: the two ventricles and atria have essentially the same diameter[15]. When compared to the aorta, the pulmonary artery is larger by 20%, while the isthmus and the ductus respectively measure only 70% and 90% of the aorta at its origin[16]. Deviations from this rule should suggest anomalies.

The biventricular shortening (a measure of the contractility) ranges from 23 to 35%[17].

## Identification of the cardiac structures

The simplifications described earlier are not valid when examining fetuses at risk of cardiac anomalies since they may have dextrocardia or ventricular inversion. A stricter method of identification uses the following *intrinsic* criteria.

### Recognition of the atria

(1) 'The atria follows the viscera': this dictum refers to the fact that there is a close relationship between the ontogenesis of the heart and that of the thoracic and abdominal organs. For the fetal sonologist, the most relevant observation is that the right atrium is always on the same side of the inferior vena cava. Evaluation of the topography of the other abdominal organs is also of value, albeit to a lesser degree. Indeed, the position of the stomach pre-

dicts the side of the left atrium, but only *as long as the fetus does not have heterotaxy*. The position of the atria can be inferred from the bronchial anatomy. While we cannot assess the bronchus, it is sometimes possible to recognize a left lung from a right lung. When a pleural effusion (common in non-immune hydrops) dissects between the lobes, the number of fissures (one on the left lung, two on the right lung) can be counted.

(2) The pulmonary veins drain into the left atrium, with the important exception of anomalous venous return.

(3) The foramen ovale flap beats towards the left atrium, with the exception of mitral atresia, in which the flap herniates in the right atrium.

### Recognition of the ventricles

(1) The left ventricle has a smoother inner surface than the right ventricle, but this is difficult to recognize.

(2) *The valves follow the ventricle;* thus a bicuspid valve is an indicator of a left ventricle, while a tricuspid valve marks a right ventricle.

(3) There are only two papillary muscles in the left ventricle, three in the right ventricle.

(4) The right ventricle has a prominent papillary muscle in its apex called the *moderator band*.

(5) The tricuspid valve inserts on the interventricular septum closer to the apex than the mitral valve.

(6) Papillary muscles insert on the septum only on the right ventricle.

## What do you mean, you can't see all that?

Neither can we. At least not in every fetus. You should be able to see the four-chamber view in 99% and the short-axis view in 70%[18]. There are, unfortunately, no special tricks except for good spatial orientation, good hand–eye co-ordination, good equipment and patience. Practice is what will make you successful. The common refrain that 'We do not do enough cardiac anomalies to be good at it' is not a good excuse. The first step is to detect that an anomaly is present. Then, the patient can be referred to a center with special expertise, which is necessary not only for a proper diagnosis, but also for counselling the couple with regard to the fetal prognosis.

## M-MODE

Since the fetal echocardiogam is difficult to derive, one uses the M-mode recording to deduce from the mechanical events the electrical signal that caused them. In M-mode ultrasound, one line of information only is continuously displayed: instead of a two-dimensional scan of the heart, a recording of the variations of echoes along a single line is produced. Thus, M-mode is of little help in the analysis of the morphology of the heart but is useful in assessing motions and rhythms. Historically, M-mode was just recorded with a pencil-like transducer, and orientation was a major problem. Current equipment displays a two-dimensional image alongside the M-mode recording which simplifies the orientation. Most machines allow toggling between a display of the M-mode, the real-time or a combination of the two. The gain and magnification of the M-mode can often be set independently from that of the real-time. Since the M-mode recording is along a single line, there is no focal zone to set.

The most common use for M-mode is in documenting fetal cardiac activity. One simply 'drops' an M-mode line over the fetal heart and records the activity. The machine allows calculation of the fetal rhythm. A grid of dots is overlaid on the image. The vertical spacing of the dots is 1 cm; the horizontal spacing is 0.5 seconds. This allows evaluation of the fetal rhythm even if it was not computed at the time of the examination. If the beats are simultaneous with every horizontal marker, the rhythm is 120 per min (one every half second); if it is every two markers, 60 beats per min (bpm); and every three

markers, 40 bpm. Two beats per marker (thus 4 per second) represent a tachycardia at 240 bpm.

M-mode was also used to measure the diameters of cardiac chambers. The two-dimensional images are far easier to interpret, and M-mode is now obsolete for this application. Finally, some authors have attempted to derive other values of cardiac activity such as pre-ejection fraction, rate of fractional shortening, etc. This can safely be ignored since they have not contributed to improved diagnostic accuracy.

### Wall and septal motion

When the transducer is placed perpendicular to the interventricular septum (Figure 7), one can recognize, from top to bottom: the anterior wall and ventricle (with flashes of atrioventricular valve echoes), the septum, the distal ventricle and the posterior wall. A small amount of pericardial fluid can sometimes be seen during systole on the outside of the epicardium and medial to the bright echo that represents the

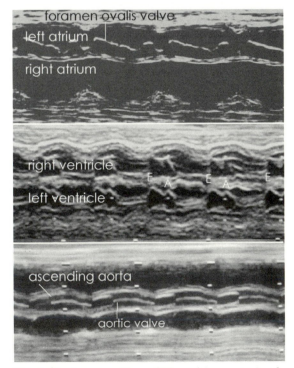

**Figure 7** A composition of M-mode sonograms obtained at various levels within the fetal heart

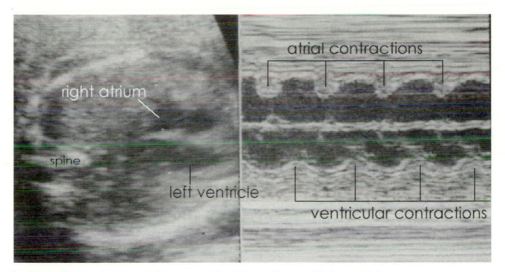

**Figure 8**    M-mode sonograms passing across the right atrium and left ventricle

pericardium[19]. Systole is marked by a nearing of the anterior and posterior walls, diastole by a separation of these echoes. Note that, in the fetus, there is minimal motion of the septum.

Which ventricle is anterior and which is posterior depends on the fetal position. In breech fetuses, the anterior ventricle is the right one when the fetus has its spine to the mother's left and the left ventricle when its spine is on the mother's right. In cephalic fetuses, the anterior ventricle is the right one when the fetus has its spine to the mother's right and the left ventricle when its spine is on the mother's left.

This biventricular M-mode is of little clinical use. A more important section is obtained by dropping the M-mode line through an atrium and a ventricle (Figure 8). In this view, the middle echoes will represent either the interventricular or interatrial septum, or an atrioventricular valve with, on either side, an atrial wall and a ventricular wall. This permits an analysis of the transmission of the impulse from the atrium to the ventricle and allows a rapid differential diagnosis of all forms of dysrhythmias.

## Foramen ovale motion

The movement of the foramen ovale is complicated. The valve opens and closes twice during the cardiac cycle. It opens for the first time during ventricular systole when returning blood cannot go through the closed tricuspid valve and passes through the foramen ovale toward the left atrium. At the beginning of the diastole, the tricuspid valve opens, thus releasing the pressure, and the foramen ovale valve closes. The opening of the atrioventricular valve is soon followed by contraction of the atria. This pushes blood from the right atrium into the left and opens the foramen ovale for the second time. The valve then closes for the second time at the end of the atrial kick. Thus, there will be two periods of opening: a long one during diastole and a short one during systole (Figure 7).

## Valvular motion

### The mitral and tricuspid valves

The anterior leaflet of the mitral valve has a typical *M-shaped* motion (Figure 7). In early diastole, the rush of blood into the left ventricle rapidly opens the valve, and the leaflet moves towards the interventricular septum. After the initial filling of the ventricle, the flow slows, and the leaflet moves away from the septum. This creates a 'peak' (the E point), and the motion away from the 'peak' is called the EF segment. The atrial kick increases the flow again, pushing the leaflet towards the septum. This creates another ascending segment (FA). The leaflet closes by moving away from the septum. The initiation of the ventricular contraction causes an undulation (the B point), and then the closure of the valve. The valve remains closed until the onset of diastole (the D point). The posterior leaflet is shorter and has a smaller motion that mirrors the motion of the anterior leaflet: it moves towards the posterior wall instead of the septum.

### The aortic and pulmonary valves

The M-mode motion of the aortic valve has a typical 'box' appearance (Figure 7). The free edge of the valve is seen during diastole in the middle of the lumen of the aorta as a bisecting line. The opening of the aortic valve is very rapid. The semilunar valves move toward the aortic wall. This rapid opening describes the left side of the 'box'. The box remains open during the whole systole. An equally brisk closure forms the right side of the box. The same image can be obtained from the pulmonary valve, but is usually technically more difficult to obtain.

## Pulsed wave and color Doppler

Pulsed wave Doppler is used to analyze the *spectral shift* (to assess the resistance in a vessel), to obtain *flow velocities* (how the resistance affects the flow), and *flow predictions* (to estimate the perfusion). Measurements are obtained during fetal apnea. The spectral analysis is independent of the angle of interrogation and thus is the most operator-independent measurement. Flow velocity assumes that the angle between the ultrasound beam and the flow is correctly estimated (and less than 30°). Flow measurements add to this restriction that the exact size of the section of the vessel is known and that the flow has a flat profile (all the red cells travel at the same speed, and those on the edge of the vessel are not slower). Unfortunately, the more physiological measurements are thus the least reliable.

Adequate recordings of velocity waveforms of the blood flow through the atrioventricular valves, great vessels and inferior vena cava can be obtained in almost all cases starting from 18

to 20 weeks. Pulsed Doppler ultrasound, in combination with two-dimensional and M-mode sonography, has proved useful in the evaluation of both fetal dysrhythmias and structural anomalies.

Color Doppler overlays a representation of flow velocity over a conventional gray-scale image. This allows a rapid recognition of the flow pattern. Color Doppler is useful to assess normal anatomy and physiology[20], valvular regurgitation or stenosis, shunting and the orientation of flows to obtain the most representative pulse wave spectrum[21].

An in-depth review of the use of pulsed wave and color Doppler in the investigation of cardiac anatomy and function is provided elsewhere in this book.

We believe that, in any dedicated examination of the fetal heart, the real-time examination should be accompanied by either color or pulsed wave Doppler demonstration of blood flow across the atrioventricular and semilunar valves.

## THE STEP-BY-STEP ANALYSIS

A systematic approach to the heart simplifies its study. The approach widely used by pathologists or pediatric cardiologists relies on the identification of the left and right atria, ventricles and great vessels. This is unfortunately rarely feasible in the fetus since the heart is too small and the resolution insufficient to detect the identifying criteria. Structures such as the atrial appendages or bronchus are essentially invisible in the fetus, especially before 24 weeks. Furthermore, common clues such as the presence of cyanosis and pulmonary overcirculation simply do not exist in the fetus.

The following approach is a derivative of the pathologist's approach, adapted to what can be recognized in the fetus. It starts with the identification of readily recognizable landmarks and progresses to more subtle findings. The step-by-step approach that we use reviews the identification of the fetal position, the position of the heart in relation to the body, the number of chambers and their connections, and finally the rhythms. Before that, we must review the criteria used to identify the cardiac structures.

## Fetal and cardiac position

To assess the cardiac situs, observe the fetal position: is it cephalic or breech? Then identify the cardiac apex. This usually does not present any problem. Finally, assess the position of the aortic arch and that of the stomach; both should be on the same side as the cardiac apex. The descending aorta can be seen slightly on the side of the spine. When in doubt about its position, mentally divide the fetal chest in two equal halves by a line that traverses the middle of the vertebra. The aorta should be on one side of this line and not be divided by it.

### The fetus in cephalic position

The fetal spine can either be on the mother's left (right of the screen) or on the mother's right (left of the screen). Remember that it is important to adhere to the standard orientation of the American Institute of Ultrasound in Medicine here: no creativity allowed until you are quite confident about what you do!

When the fetal spine is on the mother's left, the transducer is closer to the right side of the fetus than to its left side. Therefore, the stomach, apex and aortic arch ought to be on the 'far side' of the fetus (away from the transducer): this is situs solitus. If they are on the proximal side the fetus has a situs inversus; in any other condition, the fetus has heterotaxy. On the right side, of the fetus, the inferior vena cava should be seen.

Similarly, when the fetal spine is on the mother's right, the transducer is closer to the left side of the fetus than to its right side. Therefore, the stomach, apex and aortic arch ought to be close to the transducer (situs solitus). If they are on the 'far side', the fetus has a situs inversus; in any other condition the fetus has heterotaxy.

### The fetus in breech position

The same reasoning applies to the breech fetus. When its spine is on the mother's left, its stomach, apex and aortic arch should be close to the transducer (situs solitus). If they are away, the fetus has situs inversus; if they are discordant, the fetus has heterotaxy.

When the spine is on the mother's right, its stomach, apex and descending aorta should be away from the transducer (situs solitus). If they are close, the fetus has situs inversus; if they are discordant, the fetus has heterotaxy.

Once the fetal position, the apex, the aortic arch, the stomach and inferior vena cava are identified, one can establish the situs. But before examining the different combinations, let us review what the usual combinations are.

## Definitions

The normal situation – cardiac apex, stomach and aortic arch on the left, inferior vena cava on the right – is called *situs solitus* (Figure 9). A mirror image of the situs solitus is called *situs inversus*. If some of the organs are on the correct side while others are on the opposite of their expected side, the situation is called *heterotaxy* or *situs ambiguus*. Heterotaxy can be divided according to which organ is abnormal, into *dextrocardia* when the heart is on the right side and the stomach on the left side, and *visceral situs* when the heart is on the left and the stomach on the right. The first condition is also referred to as *situs solitus with dextrocardia*, while the second is referred to as *situs inversus with levocardia*. When the heart and/or the viscera are not frankly on one side but tend to be midline, the condition is called *visceral heterotaxia*. Very rarely, the heart will be in a midline position. This is referred to as *mesocardia*.

Before deciding that the heart is on the 'wrong' side, one has to distinguish between two conditions that may be confused. The heart may be on the right side because the heart has an intrinsic abnormality: this is referred to as *dextrocardia*. Sometimes, however, the heart can be on the right side because of an abnormality which is extrinsic to the heart. This is called *dextroposition*. The heart is either pushed away from the left to the right by a diaphragmatic hernia, congenital lobar emphysema or a cystadenomatoid malformation of the lung or it occupies a void on the right in case of right lung agenesis.

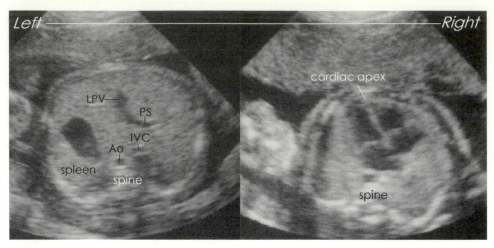

**Figure 9** The fetal situs is assessed by two cross-sections obtained at the level of the upper abdomen and chest. In the former view, under normal circumstances, the stomach, spleen, and descending aorta (Ao) are seen to the left. The left portal vein (LPV) bends to the right and connects to the portal sinus (PS). The inferior vena cava (IVC) is seen to the right and anterior to the aorta. Within the chest, the cardiac apex is oriented to the left

The determination of the situs is important since it is an important predictor of the presence of cardiac anomalies: in situs solitus the frequency of congenital anomalies is roughly 1%; in situs inversus it is doubled to 2%. Although the frequency of cardiac anomalies is low in situs solitus, situs solitus is by far the most common configuration; thus, most cardiac anomalies occur in those patients. In heterotaxy, the frequency of cardiac anomalies is considerably higher: over 75% in dextrocardia and over 95% in visceral heterotaxia. In dextrocardia, one should look for left to right shunts (atrial septal defects, anomalous venous return or ventricular septal defects) and obstruction to the right outflow (pulmonic stenosis or atresia). There is no specific prevalence of disorders in visceral heterotaxia. Congenitally corrected transposition of the great arteries is common in both visceral heterotaxia and dextrocardia and is also increased in situs inversus.

## Cardiac structures and their connections

### Great vessels and atrial connections

A section high in the mediastinum is used to assess the side of the aortic arch. One can also look for the position of the descending aorta in the high chest. This is more delicate since whichever side the aorta is on it will ultimately enter the abdomen through the esophageal hiatus and thus be almost midline. The relative position of the aorta and the vena cava should also be noted. In situs solitus and in situs inversus, the aorta and vena cava are on the contralateral side of the midline with the cava ipsilateral to the right atrium[22]. This relation is not true in atrial isomerism. In polysplenia, the cava is interrupted and continued into the hemiazygos which is ipsilateral and posterior to the aorta. In asplenia, the cava is ipsilateral and anterior to the aorta, and the hepatic vein enters the atrium independently from the cava.

### Atrioventricular connections

The following connections may exist: two atria connected to separate ventricles or to the same ventricle, or one atrium connected to a single ventricle. If the atria are connected to their respective ventricles, they are said to be *concordant*, while they are *discordant* when they connect to the opposite anatomical ventricle. When both atria connect to a single ventricle, the condition is called *double inlet* ventricle.

*Ventriculo-arterial connections*

Finally, the concordance between the ventricles and the great vessels and the position of the vessels should be assessed. Just as before, the connections are concordant when the correct ventricle is connected to the corresponding great vessel, and discordant when it is connected to the opposite vessel. When more than half of both great vessels originate from one ventricle, the situation is called *double outlet* ventricle. Finally, a *single outlet* heart corresponds to the emergence of a single great vessel from the heart: a truncus, an aorta with pulmonary atresia, or a pulmonary artery with aortic atresia.

*Rhythms*

Fetal cardiac activity is detectable from 6 weeks by suprapubic ultrasound[23] and about 1 week earlier by transvaginal ultrasound. In very early pregnancy, high-resolution vaginal sonography may demonstrate the embryo prior to the onset of cardiac activity. The normal fetal heart rate varies with gestational age. It is around 100 beats/min at 8 weeks, reaches 175 beats/min by 10 weeks, 150 at 15 weeks[24,25] and slows further to about $140 \pm 20$ beats/min at 20 weeks and $130 \pm 20$ beats/min at term[26].

When the rate is greater than 160 beats/min, one talks about tachycardia; when it is below 100, the condition is referred to as bradycardia. Short episodes of bradycardia, sometimes as slow as 50 beats/min, are probably physiological, especially in the second trimester.

The heart rate is influenced by maternal smoking[27] and maximal maternal effort[28] but not by submaximal (65%) exercise[29] or terbutalin treatment[30].

## WHEN AND WHY DO A CARDIAC EXAMINATION

### When

A full cardiac examination is a time-consuming investigation which is not recommended for every patient, at present. Unless there is a specific indication for fetal echocardiography, the standard of practice in the United States as well as in most European countries is to limit the examination to the following: fetal position, situs and a four-chamber view. This allows the detection of a large number of anomalies, not only cardiac but also gastrointestinal (diaphragmatic hernia) and pulmonary (cystic adenomatoid malformation, lung agenesis)[31]. The rest of the investigation belongs to the dedicated cardiac examination[5]. Cardiac examinations are easiest to perform between 20 and 24 weeks. Earlier examinations are more difficult because of the small size of the heart; later examinations are impaired by increasing calcification of the shoulders, arms and ribs. The use of vaginal sonography in very early gestation is described elsewhere in this book.

### Why

Dedicated examinations (often called 'fetal echo' or 'echocardiography') are performed for familial/maternal or fetal reasons[32]. The result of the examination will affect the prenatal care in several ways. When the examination is normal, the parent can be reassured – with the *caveat* that some anomalies can still be overlooked. Some of the tachyarrhythmias can be treated *in utero*. When the anomaly is treatable, delivery in a tertiary care center familiar with the treatment of congenital heart disease should be encouraged. When a lethal anomaly is discovered, interruption of the pregnancy can be offered or, when after the legal limit of termination, non-interventional obstetric care given.

*Familial reasons*

Familial reasons include a sibling with or a history of cardiac anomaly, maternal diabetes, toxic exposure (drugs, medications, alcohol, etc.), and infections. The recurrence rate of cardiac anomalies is 2% overall, but some anomalies such as hypoplastic left heart syndrome, coarctation of the aorta and the cardiosplenic syndromes may have a recurrence rate as high as 10%[33] (Table 1). Table 2 lists some of the cardiac anomalies in the offspring of mothers exposed

**Table 1** Recurrence risks (%) of congenital heart disease

| | Recurrence risks | | |
|---|---|---|---|
| Defect | One sibling affected[47] | Father affected[48] | Mother affected[49] |
| Aortic stenosis | 2 | 3 | 13–18 |
| Atrial septal defect | 2.5 | 5 | 4–4.5 |
| Atrioventricular canal | 2 | 1 | 14 |
| Coarctation | 2 | 2 | 4 |
| Patent ductus arteriosus | 3 | 2.5 | 3.5–4 |
| Pulmonary stenosis | 2 | 2 | 4–6.5 |
| Tetralogy of Fallot | 2.5 | 1.5 | 2.5 |
| Ventricular septal defect | 3 | 2 | 6–10 |

to certain drugs or disease. The number of cases reported in the literature is immensely greater, but few of the reports allow differentiation between a coincidental association and a true statistical relation[34]. Those listed are those thought to have a statistical relation.

*Fetal indications*

Fetal indications include:

*Signs of trisomy (13, 18, 21)*   Search for endocardial cushion defect, atrial septal defect, ventricular septal defect, tetralogy of Fallot, double outlet right ventricle, univentricular heart, truncus, transposition of the great vessels, hypoplastic left heart syndrome and tricuspid atresia, among others[35].

*Hydrops or polyhydramnios*   This is a very typical association that suggests circulatory failure. The causes of circulatory failure include:

(1)  Obstructive diseases such as malformations (aortic atresia, calcinosis, etc.), torsion of the great vessels by an extracardiac mass (cystic adenomatoid tumor of the lung, cardiac teratoma or diaphragmatic hernia);

(2)  Arrhythmias (either bradycardia or, more commonly, severe tachycardia); or

(3)  Decreased oxygen carrying capacity of the blood usually from anemia (isoimmunization, fetomaternal hemorrhage, etc.) or other causes (increased blood viscosity in the recipient twin of a twin-to-twin transfusion).

*Anomaly of situs*   This suggests cardiosplenic syndromes.

*Bradycardia*   Search for an anomaly of the conducting system, either due to an absent or anomalous connection in the connecting system (atrial septal defect, endocardial cushion defect, transposition) or damage due to autoimmune reactions (maternal lupus).

*Growth retardation*   Either 'symmetrical' (think of TORCH infections or chromosomal anomalies and their associated cardiac anomalies) or 'asymmetrical' growth retardation[36] is associated with cardiac anomalies.

*Cystic hygroma*   This should suggest Turner syndrome and thus coarctation of the aorta and hypoplastic left heart syndrome.

*Vertebral anomalies*   Search for anomalies of the VACTERL association (ventricular septal defect) or Klippel–Feil syndrome (atrial septal defect, coarctation).

*Sacral meningoceles*   These have also been associated with conotruncal anomalies[37].

*Hand and feet anomalies*   Numerous syndromes associated with acromelic and cardiac anomalies.

*First branchial arch anomalies*   Mandible and lower facial anomalies are associated with conotruncal anomalies (great vessel anomalies)[38].

**Table 2** Maternal medications and disorders and cardiac anomalies

| | | | |
|---|---|---|---|
| *Alcohol*[49]<br>atrial septal defect<br>ventricular septal defect<br>endocardial cushion<br>  defect<br>pulmonary aplasia<br>tetralogy of Fallot | tetralogy of Fallot<br>double outlet right<br>  ventricle<br>atrial septal defect<br>Ebstein's anomaly | *Trimethobenzamide*[60]<br>various<br><br>*Vitamin A*[61]<br>various | *Lupus*[67]<br>congenital heart block<br>atrial septal defect<br>pulmonary stenosis |
| *Anticonvulsants*[50,51]<br>ventricular septal defect<br>tetralogy of Fallot<br>atrial septal defect<br>aortic stenosis<br>transposition of the<br>  great arteries | *Indomethacin*[54]<br>premature closure of<br>  the ductus<br><br>*Lithium*[55]<br>coarctation of the aorta<br>tricuspid regurgitation<br>atrial flutter<br>Ebstein's anomaly<br>pulmonary atresia | *Coxsackie B virus*[62]<br>myocarditis<br><br>*Cytomegalovirus*[63]<br>tetralogy of Fallot<br><br>*Diabetes*[64]<br>transposition of great<br>  arteries<br>ventricular septal defect<br>coarctation of the aorta<br>atrial septal defect<br>endocardial cushion<br>  defect<br>left heart hypoplasia | *Mumps*[68]<br>endocardial<br>  fibroelastosis<br><br>*Phenylketonuria*[69]<br>ventricular septal defect<br>coarctation of the aorta<br>tetralogy of Fallot<br>pulmonary atresia<br>pulmonary stenosis |
| *Antineoplastics*<br>tetralogy of Fallot | *Phenothiazines*[56]<br>various | | *Rubella*[70,71]<br>atrial septal defect<br>ventricular septal defect<br>tricuspid valve atresia<br>pulmonary stenosis<br>pulmonary valve<br>  stenosis<br>aortic valve stenosis<br>aortic arch anomalies<br>coarctation of the aorta<br>Ebstein's anomaly |
| *Barbiturates*[52]<br>ventricular septal defect<br>coarctation of the aorta<br>pulmonary stenosis | *Prochlorperazine*[52]<br>ventricular septal defect | | |
| *Chlorotheophylline*[52]<br>various | *Salicylates*[57,58]<br>atrial septal defect<br>left heart hypoplasia<br>ventricular septal defect | *Epilepsy*[65]<br>transposition of great<br>  arteries<br>atrial septal defect<br>tetralogy of Fallot<br>coarctation of the aorta | |
| *Exogenous female sexual<br>hormones*[53]<br>ventricular septal defect<br>aortic stenosis<br>tricuspid atresia<br>patent ductus arteriosus<br>transposition of great<br>  arteries | *Thalidomide*[59]<br>ventricular septal defect<br>atrial septal defect<br>tetralogy of Fallot<br>truncus arteriosus<br>  communis<br>pulmonary stenosis | *Hyperphenylalaninemia*[66]<br>ventricular septal defect<br>atrial septal defect<br>tetralogy of Fallot | *Toxoplasmosis*[63]<br>myocarditis<br>aortic stenosis<br>ventricular septal defect |

*Single umbilical artery* Numerous anomalies have been reported including: atrial septal defect, ventricular septal defect, hypoplastic ventricle, tetralogy of Fallot, truncus, transposition, anomalous pulmonary venous return, coarctation, dextrocardia.

*Persistent right umbilical vein* Occasionally associated with a variety of cardiac defects.

*Extracardiac anomalies* Cardiac anomalies are associated with extracardiac anomalies in 5–10%. Conversely, non-cardiac anomalies occur in 7–17% of fetuses with a cardiac anomaly[39]. Because of these associations, we perform a cardiac echo and karyotype for every fetus in which an anomaly is found.

## FREQUENCY OF CARDIAC ANOMALIES

Congenital heart diseases occur in about 0.6% of newborns. The distribution of anomalies detected in fetuses is strongly biased toward the more severe anomalies. When stillborn and early fetal deaths are included, the number of anomalies rises. Approximately 5% of the defects are associated with chromosomal defects in the pediatric population, while in the fetal groups the frequency rises to 40% when the anomaly is detected around 20 weeks[40] and decreases to 13% close to term, with an overall risk of 25%[15]. By far the most common aneuploidy is trisomy 21 (89%) followed by trisomy 18 and 13 (4% each) and Turner syndrome (1%). Two per cent of cardiac anomalies are associated with environmental factors. The recurrence risk after the birth of one affected child is 2–5% and 10% after the birth of two affected siblings[41].

## RELIABILITY OF PRENATAL DIAGNOSIS

The accuracy of prenatal diagnosis is difficult to establish[42]. It is certain that numerous excellent diagnoses have been made prenatally; however, an exact match between the prenatal and the pathological diagnoses is very difficult to achieve since prenatal examination often misses some of the more subtle and accessory findings[43]. We are very suspicious of the accuracy reported in some series, and we agree that only about half of the anomalies are detected[44]. By including just a few differential diagnoses in the report, the likelihood of including the correct one easily reaches 75%, thus giving falsely good results.

The number of anomalies that are missed is even harder to estimate. Prenatal echocardiography has a tendency to detect the more severe anomalies (univentricular heart, tricuspid atresia, endocardial cushion defects) and miss the more benign anomalies (atrial septal defect, patent ductus arteriosus, etc.). Lesions that have commonly been missed include ventricular septal defect (membranous and muscular), secundum atrial septal defect, coarctation, supravalvar aortic stenosis and tetralogy of Fallot[45] among others. Lesions that affect the four-chamber view are more commonly detected than conotruncal lesions. Finally, the natural evolution of some anomalies may be such that they only appear in the third trimester and are absent earlier.

In a high-risk population of 1577 fetuses with a slightly enriched number of anomalies (1.8% instead of 0.6%), the *sensitivity* of prenatal ultrasound to detect fetuses with cardiac anomalies is 62%, the *specificity* (correct identification of fetuses without anomaly) is 100%, the *positive predictive value* (the likelihood of a correct prediction of anomaly) 100%, and the *negative predictive value* (the likelihood of a correct prediction of absence of anomaly) 99%. In fetuses identified as having an anomaly of any organ system, the likelihood of a cardiac anomaly increases to 7.5%. The sensitivity is 96%, specificity 99%, positive predictive value 95% and negative predictive value 99%[46].

# References

1. Rudolph, A. M. (1985). Distribution and regulation of blood flow in the fetal and neonatal lamb. *Circul. Res.*, **57**, 811–21
2. Pearson, A. A. and Sauter, R. W. (1971). Observation on the phrenic nerves and the ductus venosus in human embryos and fetuses. *Am. J. Obstet. Gynecol.*, **110**, 560–5
3. Rabischong, P. and Dayan, L. (1965). Etude anatomique et fonctionnelle de l'evolution du canal d'Arantius. *Bull. Assoc. Anat.*, **128**, 1342–58
4. Walker, A. M. (1984). Physiological control of the fetal cardiovascular system. In Beard, R. W. and Nathanielsz, P. W. (eds.) *Fetal Physiology and Medicine* 2nd edn, pp. 287–316. (New York: Marcel Dekker Inc)
5. Cyr, D. R., Guntheroth, W. G., Mack, L. A. *et al.* (1986). A systematic approach to fetal echocardiography using real time/two dimensional sonography. *J. Ultrasound Med.*, **5**, 343–50
6. Klinkenbijl, J. and Wenink, A. C.(1988). Morphology of sections through the fetal heart. *Int. J. Cardiol.*, **20**, 87–98
7. Allan, L. D., Crawford, D. C., Chita, S. K. *et al.* (1986). Prenatal screening for congenital heart disease. *Br. Med. J.*, **292**, 1717–9
8. Comstock, C. H. (1987). Normal fetal heart axis and position. *Obstet. Gynecol.*, **70**, 255–9
9. Benbow, E. W., Love, E. M., Love, H. G. *et al.* (1987). Massive right atrial thrombus associated with a Chiari network and a Hickman catheter. *Am. J. Clin. Pathol.*, **88**, 243–8
10. Jeanty, P., Romero, R., Cantraine, F. *et al.* (1984). Fetal cardiac dimensions: a potential tool for the diagnosis of congenital heart defects. *J. Ultrasound Med.*, **3**, 359–64
11. De Vore, G. R. (1984). Fetal echocardiography a new frontier. *Clin. Obstet. Gynecol.*, **27**, 359–77
12. Veille, J. C., Sivakoff, M. and Nemeth, M. (1988). Accuracy of echocardiography measurements in

the fetal lamb. *Am. J. Obstet. Gynecol.*, **158**(5), 1225–32

13. De Vore, G. R., Siassi, B. and Platt, L. D. (1985). Fetal echocardiography: V M-mode measurements of the aortic root and aortic valve in second and third trimester normal human fetuses. *Am. J. Obstet. Gynecol.*, **152**, 543–50

14. Sorensen, K. (1985). Intraobserver reperformance reproducibility of fetal echocardiographic measurements. *J. Cardiovasc. Ultr.*, **4**, 239–42

15. Allan, L. D. (1988). Fetal echocardiography. *Clin. Obstet. Gynecol.*, **31**, 61–79

16. Angelini, A., Allan, L., Anderson, R. H. *et al.* (1988). Measurements of the dimensions of the aortic and pulmonary pathways in the human fetus: a correlative echocardiographic and morphometric study. *Br. Heart J.*, **60**, 221–6

17. Wladimiroff, J. W. and McGhie, J. S. (1981). M-mode ultrasonic assessment of fetal cardiovascular dynamics. *Br. J. Obstet. Gynaecol.*, **88**, 1241–5

18. Cyr, D. R., Komarniski, C. A., Guntheroth, W. G. *et al.* (1988). The prevalence of imaging fetal cardiac anatomy. *J. Diag. Med. Sonogr.*, **6**, 299–304

19. Jeanty, P., Romero, R. and Hobbins, J. C. (1984). Fetal pericardial fluid: a normal finding of the second half of gestation. *Am. J. Obstet. Gynecol.*, **149**, 529–32

20. Redel, D. A. (1986). Doppler flow imaging: a method for displaying blood flow within the cardiovascular system. *New Dev. Imag.*, **2**, 135–40

21. Kurjak, A., Alfirevic, Z. and Miljan, M. (1988). Conventional and color Doppler in the assessment of fetal and maternal circulation. *Ultrasound Med. Biol.*, **14**, 354–77

22. Huhta, J. C., Smallhorn, J. F. and Macartney, F. J. (1982). Cross-sectional echocardiographic diagnosis of situs. *Br. Heart J.*, **48**, 388–403

23. Cadkin, A. V. and McAlpin, J. (1984). Detection of fetal cardiac activity between 41 and 43 days of gestation. *J. Ultrasound Med.*, **3**, 499–503

24. Hertzberg, B. S., Mahony, B. S. and Bowie, J. D. (1988). First trimester fetal cardiac activity. Sonographic documentation of a progressive early rise in heart rate. *J. Ultrasound Med.*, **7**, 573–5

25. Laboda, L. A., Estroff, J. A. and Benacerraf, B. R. (1989). First trimester bradycardia, a sign of impending fetal loss. *J. Ultrasound Med.*, **8**, 561–3

26. Allan, L. D., Anderson, R. H., Sullivan, I. D. *et al.* (1988). Evaluation of fetal arrhythmias by echocardiography. *Br. Heart J.*, **50**, 240–5

27. Sorensen, K. E. and Borlum, K. G. (1987). Acute effects of maternal smoking on human fetal heart function. *Acta Obstet. Gynecol. Scand.*, **66**, 217–20

28. Carpenter, M. W., Sady, S. P., Hoegsberg, B. *et al.* (1988). Fetal heart rate response to maternal exertion. *J. Am. Med. Assoc.*, **259**, 3006–9

29. Sorensen, K. E. and Borlum, K. G. (1986). Fetal heart function in response to short term maternal exercise. *Br. J. Obstet. Gynaecol.*, **93**, 310–13

30. Sorensen, K. E. and Borlum, K. G. (1988). Fetal cardiac function in response to long-term maternal terbutalin treatment. *Acta Obstet. Gynecol. Scand.*, **67**, 105–7

31. Hegge, F. N., Lees, M. H. and Watson, P. T. (1987). Utility of a screening examination of the fetal cardiac position and four-chambers during obstetric sonography. *J. Reprod. Med.*, **32**, 353–8

32. Kleinman, C. S. and Santulli, T. V. Jr (1983). Ultrasonic evaluation of the fetal human heart. *Semin. Perinatol.*, **7**, 90–101

33. Allan, L. D. (1989). Diagnosis of fetal cardiac abnormality. *Arch. Dis. Child.*, **64**, 964–8

34. Pexieder, T. (1987). Teratogens. In Pierpont, M. E. and Moller, J. H. (eds.). *The Genetics of Cardiovascular Disease* pp. 25–68 (Boston: Martinus Nijhoff Publishing)

35. Rizzo, N., Pittalis, M. C., Pilu, G., Orsini, L. F., Perolo, A. and Bovicelli, L. (1990). Prenatal karyotyping in malformed fetuses. *Prenat. Diagn.*, **10**, 17–21

36. Stewart, P. A., Wladimiroff, J. W. and Essed, C. E. (1983). Prenatal ultrasound diagnosis of congenital heart disease associated with intrauterine growth retardation. A report of 2 cases. *Prenat. Diagn.*, **3**, 279–85

37. Kousseff, B. G. (1984). Sacral meningocele with conotruncal heart defects: a possible autosomal recessive trait. *Pediatrics*, **74**, 395–8

38. Greenberg, F., Gresik, M. V., Carpenter, R. J. *et al.* (1989). The Gardner–Silengo–Wachtel or genito–palato–cardiac syndrome: male pseudohermaphroditism with micrognathia, cleft palate, and conotruncal cardiac defect. *Am. J. Med. Genet.*, **26**, 59–64

39. Copel, J. A., Pilu, G. and Kleinman, C. S. (1986). Congenital heart disease and extra-cardiac malformations. Associations and indications for fetal echocardiography. *Am. J. Obstet. Gynecol.*, **154**, 1121–7

40. Copel, J. A., Cullen, M., Green, J. J. *et al.* (1988). The frequency of aneuploidy in prenatally diagnosed congenital heart disease: an indication for fetal karyotyping. *Am. J. Obstet. Gynecol.*, **158**, 409–13

41. Nora, J. J., McGill, C. W. and McNamara, D. G. (1970). Empiric recurrence risks in common and uncommon congenital heart lesions. *Teratology*, **3**, 325–30

42. Sandor, G. G., Farquarson, D., Wittmann, B. *et al.* (1986). Fetal echocardiography: results in high risk patients. *Obstet. Gynecol.*, **67**, 358–64

43. Allan, L. D. (1985). Fetal echocardiography: confidence limits and accuracy, *editorial. Pediatr. Cardiol.*, **6**, 145–6

44. Benacerraf, B. R., Pober, B. R. and Sanders, S. P. (1987). Accuracy of fetal echocardiography. *Radiology*, **165**, 847–9

45. Todros, T., Presbitero, P., Gaglioti, P. *et al.* (1988). Pulmonary stenosis with intact ventricular septum: documentation of development of the lesion echographically during fetal life. *Int. J. Cardiol.*, **19**, 355–60

46. Stewart, P. A. (1989). Echocardiography in the human fetus. PhD thesis, Erasmus Hospital Rotterdam, Netherland, p. 62 and p. 90

47. Nora, J. J. and Nora, A. H. (1978). *Genetics and Counselling in Cardiovascular Disease.* (Springfield: Charles C. Thomas)

48. Nora, J. J. and Nora, A. H. (1987). Maternal transmission of congenital heart disease: new recurrence risk figures and the questions of cytoplasmic inheritance and vulnerability to teratogens. *Am. J. Cardiol.*, **59**, 459–64

49. Loser, H. (1981). Human alcohol embryopathy and changes at the cardiovascular system. *Teratology*, **24**, 29A–30A

50. Starreveld-Zimmerman, A. A. E., Van der Kolk, W. J., Elshove, J. and Meinardi, H. (1974). Teratogenicity of antiepileptic drugs. *Clin. Neurol. Neurosurg.*, **2**, 81–95

51. Meyer, J. G. (1973). The teratological effects of anticonvulsants and the effects on pregnancy and birth. *Eur. Neurol.*, **10**, 179–90

52. Heinonen, O. P., Slone, D. and Shapiro, S. (1977). *Birth Defects and Drugs in Pregnancy.* (Littleton: Publ. Sci. Group)

53. Heinonen, O. P., Slone, D., Monson, R. R., Hook, E. B. and Shapiro, S. (1977). Cardiovascular birth defects and antenatal exposure to female sex hormones. *N. Engl. J. Med.*, **296**, 67–9

54. Csaba, I. F., Sulyok, E. and Ertl, T. (1978). Relationship of maternal treatment with indomethacin to persistence of fetal circulation syndrome. *J. Pediatr.*, **92**, 484–5

55. Allan, L. D., Desai, G. and Tynan, M. J. (1981). Prenatal echocardiographic screening for Ebstein's anomaly for mothers on lithium therapy. *Lancet*, **2**, 875–6

56. Slone, D., Siskind, V., Heinonen, O. P. *et al.* (1977). Antenatal exposure to phenothiazines in relation to congenital malformations, perinatal mortality rate, birth weight and intelligence quotient score. *Am. J. Obstet. Gynecol.*, **128**, 386–8

57. Turner, G. and Collins, E. (1975). Fetal effects of regular salicylate ingestion in pregnancy. *Lancet*, **2**, 338–9

58. McNiel, J. R. and Dodge, F. (1973). The possible teratogenic effect of salicylates on the developing fetus. *Clin. Pediatr.*, **12**, 347–50

59. Pliess, G. (1962). Thalidomide and congenital abnormalities. *Lancet*, **1**, 1128–9

60. Milkovich, L. and Van den Berg, B. J. (1976). An evaluation of the teratogenicity of certain antinauseant drugs. *Am. J. Obstet. Gynecol.*, **125**, 244–8

61. Hussain, M. A. (1977). Nutrient reserve in congenital malformations. *Bangladesh Med. Res. Counc. Bull.*, **3**, 94–100

62. Overall, J. C. (1972). Intrauterine virus infections and congenital heart disease. *Am. Heart J.*, **84**, 828–33

63. Wagner, H. R. (1981). Cardiac disease in congenital infections. *Clin. Perinatol.*, **8**, 481–97

64. Rowland, T. W., Hubbell, J. P. and Nadas, A. S. (1973). Congenital heart disease in infants of diabetic mothers. *J. Pediatr.*, **83**, 815–20

65. Monson, R. R., Heinonen, O. P., Shapiro, S. and Slone, D. (1974). Diphenylhydantoin and epilepsy in relation to congenital malformations and mental development. *Am. J. Epidemiol.*, **100**, 509

66. Lipson, A., Beuhler, B., Bartley, J., Walsh, D., Yu, Y., O'Halloran, M. and Webster, W. (1984). Maternal hyperphenylalaninemia fetal effects. *J. Pediatr.*, **104**, 216–20

67. Chameides, L., Truex, R. C., Vetter, V., Rashkind, W. J., Galioto, F. M. and Noonan, J. A. (1977). Association of maternal systemic lupus erythematosus and congenial complete heart block. *N. Engl. J. Med.*, **297**, 1204–7

68. Dumont, M. (1978). Mumps during pregnancy. *Nouv. Presse Med.*, **7**, 4302

69. Lenke, R. R. and Levy, H. L. (1980). Maternal phenylketonuria and hyperphenylalaninemia: an international survey of the outcome of untreated and treated pregnancies. *N. Engl. J. Med.*, **303**, 1202–8

70. Jespersen, C. S., Littauer, J. and Sagild, U. (1977). Measles as a cause of fetal defects. *Acta Paediatr. Scand.*, **66**, 367–72

71. Hardy, J. (1971). Rubella as a teratogen. *Birth Defects*, **7**, 64–71

# Experimentally altered hemodynamics in the chick embryo

3

*M. L. A. Broekhuizen, J. W. Wladimiroff and A. C. Gittenberger-de Groot*

## INTRODUCTION

In the Netherlands, approximately 1500 infants with a cardiac anomaly are born each year. Insight into the mechanisms which relate structure and function during cardiovascular development may help to define etiologies of congenital heart disease. Classically, the understanding of the development of the heart and great vessels is based on collections of normal embryos and, incidentally, abnormal hearts from infants who died before or following surgery. Based on data from these abnormal hearts, and from available normal embryonic and fetal hearts, theories were developed to explain the pathogenesis of cardiac lesions. Although these studies have direct relevance for clinical management, the etiology of congenital cardiac anomalies with particular emphasis on the interaction between hemodynamics and morphology cannot be extracted from these observations.

It is obvious that flow, blood pressure and heart rate have implications for the intricate relationship of form and function[1]. Micro-Doppler and micro-pressure studies in normal chick embryos have provided valuable information on its relationship[2]. Morphologically abnormal hearts from embryonic chicks are necessary to obtain a comparable insight into the hemodynamics in abnormal cardiac development. Spontaneous anomalies, however, do not provide the necessary reproducible sequence of stages for these hemodynamic studies. To study the interaction between hemodynamics and morphology in abnormal heart development, an animal model with specific and reproducible cardiac malformations is needed. We recently developed a standardized method, using all-*trans* retinoic acid, for inducing a spectrum of outflow tract anomalies, in particular double outlet right ventricle, in the chick embryo[3].

## RETINOIC ACID MODEL

A number of investigators have tried to induce congenital anomalies of the heart either by mechanical interference with blood flow[4,5], or by application of known teratogens at different stages of development[6,7].

Our standardized method for inducing specific and reproducible cardiac anomalies used a relatively easy and non-traumatic approach, namely applying all-*trans* retinoic acid on the vitelline membrane of the chick embryo in the early stages of development. All-*trans* retinoic acid is a well-known teratogen for this purpose[8–14]. Fertilized White Leghorn chick eggs were incubated (blunt end up) at 38°C and staged according to Hamburger and Hamilton[15]. The material was subdivided into groups of embryos treated with a solution of all-*trans* retinoic acid and the solvent dimethylsulfoxide, embryos treated with only the solvent (sham-operated embryos) and control embryos.

At stage 15 (day 2½ of a 21-day incubation), each embryo, with the exception of the controls, was exposed by creating a window in the shell followed by removal of the overlying membranes. A solution containing 1.0 µg all-*trans* retinoic acid or only the solvent 2% dimethyl-sulfoxide was then deposited on the vitelline membrane of the embryo using a Hamilton syringe.

Following administration of the solution containing retinoic acid, the window was sealed with tape and the egg reincubated. Embryos were removed at stage 34 (day 8) and processed for histological sectioning in a routine way by fixing in Bouin and embedding in paraffin. Thereafter, the embryos, including the hearts, were serially sectioned. The sections were 5 μm thick and stained with Mayer's hematoxylin/eosin.

In the normal heart of a chick embryo, the pulmonary orifice is usually positioned in front of and to the left of the aortic orifice. The ascending aorta is very short, the aortic arch and the right and left brachiocephalic artery originating directly distal to the aortic orifice (Figure 1a). However, the majority of hearts of retinoic acid-treated embryos show a spectrum of a rightward shift of the aorta with and without ventricular septal defect. The rightward positioned aorta is still connected to the left ventricle in cases without ventricular septal defect, and classified as having no septation abnormalities. The presence of a ventricular septal defect in combination with the rightward positioned aorta is classified as double outlet right ventricle (Figure 1b).

## HEMODYNAMICS

Mean dorsal aortic blood flow velocities are measured with a 20 MHz pulsed Doppler velocity meter (model 545C-4 Bioengineering, University of Iowa). This equipment is validated to be accurate above 5 mm/s. The Doppler probe consists of a 750 μm piezoelectric crystal that is positioned at a 45° angle to the dorsal aorta at the level of the sinus venosus. The internal diameter of the dorsal aorta is measured at the same level with a filar micrometer eyepiece

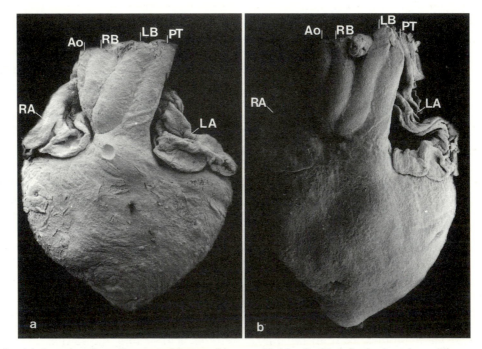

**Figure 1** (a) Anterior view of a normal heart of a stage 34 (day 8 of incubation) embryo. The great vessels are in the normal position as viewed by scanning electronmicroscopy, × 30 (RA, right atrium; Ao, aorta; RB, right brachiocephalic artery; LB, left brachiocephalic artery; PT, pulmonary trunk; LA, left atrium). (b) Anterior view of an abnormal heart of a stage 34 embryo after treatment with all-*trans* retinoic acid. The aorta and brachiocephalic arteries are displaced to the right, × 30 (RA, right atrium; Ao, aorta; RB, right brachiocephalic artery; LB, left brachiocephalic artery; PT, pulmonary trunk; LA, left atrium)

which is calibrated against a 10 μm engraved glass standard. The vessel area is calculated from the equation area $= \pi d^2/4$ where $d$ is the aortic diameter.

Blood pressure is measured in the vitelline artery with a servo-null system (model 900A, World Precision Instruments, Inc, Sarasota, Florida) and a 10 μm glass micropipette. This pressure system is validated to be accurate from $-5$ mmHg to 40 mmHg. Zero trans-tip pressure is obtained by immersing the tip of the micropipette in the extraembryonic fluid at the level of the measured site.

## Normal cardiovascular data

Hemodynamic function during rapid cardiac morphogenesis was initially defined in the dorsal aorta using a 20 MHz pulsed Doppler velocity meter in the stage 20 (day 3) to stage 35 (day 8–9) chick embryo[16]. There is a 17-fold rise in mean dorsal aortic blood flow from $0.3 \pm 0.1$ (SD) mm$^3$/s to $5.1 \pm 1.3$ (SD) mm$^3$/s. The mean heart rate doubles from $123 \pm 12$ beats/min to $239 \pm 8$ beats/min and mean stroke volume increases from $0.14 \pm 0.08$ mm$^3$ to $1.28 \pm 0.55$ mm$^3$. A stage-related rise is seen in peak systolic velocity (stage 20: $20.1 \pm 1.0$; stage 35: $82.1 \pm 7.7$ mm/s), time-averaged velocity (stage 20: $3.9 \pm 0.8$; stage 35: $19.9 \pm 4.4$ mm/s), and peak acceleration (stage 20: $687 \pm 90$; stage 35: $2506 \pm 159$ mm/s$^2$). The latter indirectly suggests an increase in cardiac contraction force.

## Altered cardiovascular data

Simultaneous measurement of dorsal aortic flow velocities and vitelline artery blood pressure together with examinations of the heart are performed in the retinoic acid model, interfering with normal cardiac development[17].

Hemodynamics of control and sham-operated embryos show no significant difference. A comparison of the hemodynamics of retinoic acid-treated embryos, control and sham-operated embryos shows a significant decrease in heart rate, peak systolic and time-averaged velocities, peak systolic and time-averaged blood flows, peak acceleration and stroke volume in retinoic acid-treated embryos. A comparison between the two subgroups of embryos treated with all-*trans* retinoic acid shows that all parameters derived from the flow velocity waveform recording are significantly reduced in the presence of a ventricular septal defect except heart rate and peak acceleration. Moreover, the dorsal aortic area, that was determined from the vessel diameter, is reduced in these embryos. Pressure readings are not essentially different between control and sham-operated embryos and all embryos treated with all-*trans* retinoic acid.

The hemodynamic changes seen in retinoic acid-treated embryos, in particular the reduced peak acceleration and stroke volume, suggest a decrease in cardiac contraction force. The peak acceleration is derived from the dorsal aortic velocity and indicates the contraction potential of the heart. Stroke volume is determined from time-averaged dorsal aortic blood flow and heart rate. The decrease in heart rate may be caused by an immature impulse formation in the conduction system due to a delay in the maturation process of the heart. Comparison between the two subgroups of retinoic acid-treated embryos reveals, in embryos with a ventricular septal defect, a significant reduction of all waveform parameters, except heart rate and peak acceleration. The latter suggests no significant difference in cardiac contraction force between the two subgroups. The abnormal morphology in combination with the decrease in cardiac contraction force could account for the impaired volume flow and could lead to the calculated reduction in vessel area in these embryos.

We propose that the hemodynamic changes are mainly due to myocardial dysfunction and to a lesser extent to abnormal cardiac morphology in embryos that are treated with all-*trans* retinoic acid. A decrease in cardiac contraction force is found in these embryos regardless of the presence of a ventricular septal defect.

Although the mechanism is unclear, we postulate that all-*trans* retinoic acid may have indirect and direct effects on the myocardium.

The indirect effect may result from an impaired parasympathetic innervation through a disturbance of the migration of cells from the neural crest. It has been reported that neural crest cells contribute to the cardiac ganglia[18,19]. Parasympathetic innervation of the heart via the cardiac ganglia could be impaired after treatment with retinoic acid. The effect of all-*trans* retinoic acid on the neural crest may be through cytotoxicity[10] or result from alterations in region-specific signals necessary for homing of neural crest cells or for their differentiation[9]. Furthermore, *in vitro* mesenchymal cell migration is inhibited by retinoids[20,21]. Impaired parasympathetic innervation could lead to an alteration of the tonus of the cardiac myocytes.

A direct effect cannot be excluded. Evidence exists that 13-*cis* retinoic acid and all-*trans* retinoic acid have multiple effects on growth and differentiation of cardiac myocytes, including an inhibition of cell proliferation, development of heart contractions, and delay in α-actin synthesis[22]. Retinoic acid may have direct effects on the myocytes by disruption of gap junctional communication[23] that could be mediated through retinoid-binding proteins[24,25] and the nuclear receptors[26]. Pexieder and colleagues[27] showed that all-*trans* retinoic acid can modify cardiac contractility. In rat fetuses treated during early pregnancy with all-*trans* retinoic acid, a higher sensitivity towards extracellular calcium ion variations was found. This could indicate a larger permeability (immaturity) of the sarcolemma and/or delayed development of the sarcoplasmic reticulum[27]. Furthermore, they reported that all-*trans* retinoic acid significantly decreased the total amount of protein in morphologically normal mouse hearts and hearts that showed a double outlet right ventricle. In these morphologically normal and abnormal hearts, the concentration of sarco-

plasmic proteins was significantly increased and that of contractile proteins decreased. Results of our study coincide with their data that, in embryos treated with all-*trans* retinoic acid complementary with structural changes of the myocardium, the function of the embryonic heart is also affected.

Both direct and indirect effects on the myocardium could generate myocardial dysfunction in various ways, and lead to the same result, i.e. a decrease in cardiac contraction force.

In conclusion, we put forward that the hemodynamic changes observed in embryos after treatment with all-*trans* retinoic acid are the result of a decrease in cardiac contraction force. Our results suggest that there is no significant difference in contraction force between the two subgroups, embryos with and without ventricular septal defect, of retinoic acid-treated embryos. The presence of a ventricular septal defect in combination with the myocardial dysfunction could account for impaired volume flow and could lead to the observed diminished dorsal aortic diameter in these embryos.

Regulation of cardiac growth and function involves the orchestration of hemodynamic and cellular events. Our model will allow us to evaluate the cellular biological aspects of the influence of all-*trans* retinoic acid on cardiac morphogenesis as well as the assessment of the hemodynamic parameters involved. This study is part of our long-term aim to obtain a better understanding into mechanisms which relate form and function during cardiovascular development. These may aid in the definition of the underlying etiologies of congenital heart disease and the optimization of clinical management.

# References

1. Clark, E. B., Hu, N., Dummett, J. L., Van de Kieft, G. K., Olson, C. and Tomanek, R. (1983). Ventricular function and morphology in chick embryo from stages 18–29. *Am. J. Physiol.*, **250**, H407–13

2. Hu, N. and Clark, E. B. (1989). Hemodynamics of stage 12 to stage 29 chick embryos. *Circulation Res.*, **65**, 1665–70

3. Broekhuizen, M. L. A., Wladimiroff, J. W., Tibboel, D., Poelmann, R. E., Wenink, A. C. G. and

Gittenberger-de Groot, A. C. (1992). Induction of cardiac anomalies with all-*trans* retinoic acid in the chick embryo. *Cardiol. Young*, **2**, 311–17

4. Colvee, E. and Hurle, J. M. (1983). Malformations of the semilunar valves produced in chick embryos by mechanical interference with cardiogenesis. *Anat. Embryol.*, **168**, 59–71

5. Rychter, Z. (1962). Experimental morphology of the aortic arches and the heart loop in the chick embryo. *Adv. Morphogen.*, **2**, 333–71

6. Loeber, C. P., Hendrix, M. J. C., Pinos de, S. D. and Golberg, S. J. (1988). Trichlorethylene: a cardiac teratogen in developing chick embryos. *Pediatr. Res.*, **24**, 740–3

7. Pexieder, T. (1986). Teratogens. In Pierpont, M. E. and Moller, J. H. (eds.) *Genetics of Cardiovascular Disease*. (Martinus Nijhoff)

8. Chytil, F. (1984). Retinoic acid: biochemistry, pharmacology, toxicology and therapeutic use. *Pharm. Rev.*, **36**, 935–45

9. Hart, R. C., McCue, P. A., Ragland, W. L., Winn, K. J. and Unger, E. R. (1990). Avian model for 13-*cis*-retinoic acid embryopathy: demonstration of neural crest related defects. *Teratology*, **41**, 463–72

10. Jellinek, R. and Kistler, A. (1981). Effect of retinoic acid upon the chick embryonic morphogenetic systems. The embryotoxicity range. *Teratology*, **23**, 191–5

11. Kawashima, H., Ohno, I., Ueno, Y., Nakaya, S., Kato, E. and Taniguchi, N. (1987). Syndrome of microtia and aortic arch anomalies resembling isoretinoin embryopathy. *J. Pediatr.*, **111** (5), 738–40

12. Lammer, E. J., Chen, D. T., Hoa, R. M., Agnish, W. D., Benke, P. J., Curry, C. J., Fernhoff, P. M., Grix, A. W., Lott, I. T., Richard, J. M. and Sun, S. C. (1985). Retinoic acid embryopathy. *N. Engl. J. Med.*, **313**, 837–41

13. Rosa, F. W., Wil, A. L. and Kelsey, F. O. (1986). Teratogen update. Vitamin A congeners. *Teratology*, **33**, 355–64

14. Yasuda, Y., Okamoto, M., Konishi, H., Matsuo, T., Kihara, T. and Tanimura, T. (1986). Developmental anomalies induced by all-*trans* retinoic acid in fetal mice: 1. Macroscopic findings. *Teratology*, **34**, 37–49

15. Hamburger, V. and Hamilton, H. L. (1951). A series of normal stages in the development of the chick embryo. *J. Morphol.*, **88**, 49–92

16. Broekhuizen, M. L. A., Mast, F., Struijk, P. C., Van der Bie, W., Mulder, P. G. H., Gittenberger-de Groot, A. C. and Wladimiroff, J. W. (1993). Hemodynamic parameters of stage 20 to stage 35 chick embryo. *Pediatr. Res.*, **34**, 44–6

17. Broekhuizen, M. L. A., Bouman, H. G. A., Mast, F., Mulder, P. G. H., Gittenberger-de Groot, A. C. and Wladimiroff, J. W. (1995). Hemodynamic changes in HH stage 34 chick embryos after treatment with all-trans retinoic acid. *Pediatr. Res.*, **38**, 342–8

18. Kirby, M. L. and Stewart, D. (1983). Neural crest origin of cardiac ganglion cells in the chick embryo: identification and extirpation. *Dev. Biol.*, **97**, 433–43

19. Kirby, M. L. (1993). Cellular and molecular contributions of the cardiac neural crest to cardiovascular development. *Trends cardiovasc. Med.*, **3**, 18–23

20. Thorogood, P., Smith, L., Nicol, A., McGinty, R. and Garrod, D. (1982). Effects of vitamin A on the behavior of migratory neural crest cells *in vitro*. *J. Cell. Sci.*, **57**, 331–50

21. Smith-Thomas, L., Lott, I. and Bronner-Fraser, M. (1987). Effects of isoretinoin on the behavior of neural crest cells *in vitro*. *Dev. Biol.*, **123**, 276–80

22. Wiens, D. J., Mann, T. K., Fedderson, D. E., Rathmell, W. K. and Franck, B H. (1992). Early heart development in the chick embryo: effects of isoretinoin on cell proliferation, $\alpha$-actin synthesis, and development of contractions. *Differentiation*, **51**, 105–12

23. Mehta, P., Bertram, J. and Loewenstein, W. (1989). The actions of retinoids on cellular growth correlate with their actions on gap junctional communication. *J. Cell. Biol.*, **108**, 1053–65

24. Maden, M., Ong, D. E., Summerbell, D. and Chytil, F. (1989). The role of retinoid-binding proteins in the generation of pattern in the developing limb, the regenerating limb and the nervous system. *Development*, **107** (Supplement), 109–19

25. Maden, M., Hunt, P., Erikson, U., Kuroiwa, A., Krumlauf, R. and Summerbell, D. (1991). Retinoic acid-binding protein, rhombomeres and the neural crest. *Development*, **111**, 35–44

26. Ruberte, E., Dollé, P., Chambon, P. and Morriss-Kay, G. (1991). Retinoic acid receptors and cellular retinoid binding proteins. II. Their differential pattern of transcription during early morphogenesis in mouse embryos. *Development*, **111**, 45–60

27. Pexieder, T., Blanc, O., Pelouch, B., Ostádalová, I., Milerová, M. and Ostádal, B. (1995). Late fetal development of retinoic acid induced transposition of great arteries – morphology, physiology and biochemistry. In Markwald, R. R., Clark, E. B. and Takao, A. (eds.) *Developmental Mechanisms of Heart Disease*, pp. 297–307. (Armark, NY: Futura Publishing Company)

# First- and early second-trimester diagnosis of fetal cardiac anomalies

# 4

*U. Gembruch, A. A. Baschat, G. Knöpfle and M. Hansmann*

## INTRODUCTION

Congenital heart disease is common, occurring in 0.4–1.0% of live births[1]. The efforts of fetal cardiology focus on an earlier diagnosis of cardiac malformations to optimize management early in pregnancy and to minimize emotional and physical trauma to the parents by earlier directed counseling or early termination of pregnancy. Second-trimester echocardiography via the transabdominal route is a well-established method today. Two-dimensional echocardiography performed at referral centers for fetal echocardiography is sufficient to diagnose most congenital heart diseases from 18 weeks of gestation[2]. The additional use of color-coded Doppler gives information about the spatial and temporal distribution of blood flow and allows the discrimination of laminar and turbulent flow patterns[3,4]. As 90% of congenital heart diseases occur in an unselected 'normal' group of obstetric patients, screening for heart disease should be introduced as an integral part of the routine obstetric scan between 18 and 22 weeks of gestation[5]. These second-trimester screening programs for congenital heart diseases that are based on the four-chamber view have detection rates for cardiac defects ranging from 45% in low-risk patients to 60% in mixed collectives[6–8]. Visualization of both ventricular outflow tracts and the pulmonary artery and aorta increases the sensitivity of the examination by 20–30%. In particular, this is due to the diagnosis of outlet ventricular septal defects, double outlet right ventricle, tetralogy of Fallot, truncus arteriosus and transposition of the great arteries[6–8].

In the embryo, the development of the heart begins on day 16. First pulsation of the cardiac tube can be observed in the 5th week of gestation from the last menstrual period. Cardiac development is finished by the 10th week at an embryonic length of 40 mm. The use of high-frequency vaginal ultrasound probes with high resolution enables a detailed examination of the embryo, making first-trimester diagnosis of various malformations possible[9–11].

## VISUALIZATION OF THE NORMAL HEART

High-frequency transvaginal probes allow a detailed investigation of fetal cardiac anatomy from the 13th week of gestation onwards. When using transvaginal two-dimensional echocardiography, Johnson and colleagues[12] reported 74% and 72% success rates in visualizing the four-chamber view at 13 and 14 weeks' gestation, respectively. This could be achieved within a set time limit of 10 min. Dolkart and Reimers[13] visualized the four-chamber view in 100% of fetuses examined at 13 and 14 weeks' gestation, and in 90% at 12 weeks' gestation. Using two-dimensional echocardiography in combination with color Doppler flow imaging, we reported equal success rates of 100% at 13 and 14 weeks' gestation and 93% at 12 weeks' gestation[14] (Table 1). In contrast with the results reported by Dolkart and Reimers, who could not demonstrate the origin and crossing of the aorta with the pulmonary trunk in more than 30% of cases at 13 weeks' gestation, the demonstration of these structures was always possible in our study at 13 and 14 weeks. These results confirm that the four-chamber view can be easily demonstrated by two-dimensional echocardiography. An unfavorable fetal position with the subsequent failure to obtain the short-axis view of the great arteries ('circle and sausage view') makes for frequent difficulty in visualizing the aorta and the pulmonary artery (Color plate A). In these situations, color Doppler flow imaging facilitates identification of these vessels, increasing the success rate of transvaginal echocardiography (Color plate B). Two-dimensional echocardiography and color Doppler flow imaging complement each other as the most favorable insonation angle for B-mode is 90° and for Doppler methods 0° or 180°. However, in all studies, the concurrent visualization of the four-chamber view and great arteries was often impossible at 11 and 12 weeks' gestation, even if color Doppler flow imaging was also used.

The fetal heart doubles in size between 14 and 18 weeks and doubles again twice before term. Normative growth charts for the biometry of the heart have been published by Bronshtein and colleagues[15]. A linear correlation between fetal growth with gestational age and the growth of cardiac structures has been demonstrated. This correlation was established by measurements of the total transverse diameter of the heart, the inner diameters of the right and left ventricles, of the ascending aorta and the pulmonary trunk as measured by two-dimensional echocardiography. The total transverse cardiac diameter, for example, measured approximately 5 mm at 12 weeks', 6 mm at 13 weeks' and 7.5 mm at 14 weeks' gestation. At the same time, the ratio between transverse cardiac diameter and the transverse diameter of the chest was found to be nearly constant around 0.3 at these gestational ages.

## INTRACARDIAC BLOOD FLOW DURING EARLY PREGNANCY

Using transabdominal pulsed wave Doppler, normal values of intracardiac blood flow velocities have been established from 11 weeks of gestation onwards. At 11–12 weeks, the peak velocity during early diastolic filling of both ventricles (E-wave) is very low compared to peak velocity during atrial contraction (A-wave), resulting in an E/A ratio of approximately 0.5[16,17]. The peak E-wave velocity and the E/A ratios markedly increase with gestational age, resulting in E/A ratios ranging between 0.8 and 0.9 in late pregnancy[16,18]. This increase of the E/A ratio is associated with a concomitant dramatic decrease of percentage reverse flow in the inferior vena cava from 11 up to 20 weeks of gestation[16,17,19]. These changes suggest a shift of blood flow from late to early diastole which may be the result of increased ventricular compliance, raised ventricular relaxation rate and/or reduced afterload. In this gestational period, a physiological decrease in vascular resistance at the level of the umbilical, placental and trunk vessels is indicated by continuously increasing end-diastolic blood velocities. At the same time, there is a marked increase in the peak velocity and time velocity integral values in the pulmonary artery and ascending aorta from 11 to 20 weeks of gestation, as a consequence of increased stroke volume, raised contractility and/or reduced afterload[16–18].

**Table 1** Rate of successful visualization for the most important cardiac structures using transvaginal two-dimensional and color Doppler echocardiography[14]

| Weeks of gestation | Four-chamber view | Origin and criss-crossing of the great arteries | Both structures |
|---|---|---|---|
| 11 | 12/14 (80%) | 10/15 (67%) | 10/15 (67%) |
| 12 | 28/30 (93%) | 24/30 (80%) | 24/30 (80%) |
| 13 | 51/51 (100%) | 51/51 (100%) | 51/51 (100%) |
| 14 | 11/11 (100%) | 11/11 (100%) | 11/11 (100%) |

## DIAGNOSIS OF CARDIAC DEFECTS

To date, a complete atrioventricular canal defect with complete heart block and atrioventricular valve insufficiency has been diagnosed as early as 11 weeks + 4 days' gestation using transvaginal two-dimensional and Doppler echocardiography in 1988 and published in 1990[20]. Results of screening a group of low-risk patients for cardiac malformations by transvaginal two-dimensional echocardiography were reported by Bronshtein and colleagues[21,22] who were able to diagnose severe cardiac malformations in 47 fetuses between 12 and 16 weeks of gestation. The diagnostic efficacy of first- and early second-trimester echocardiography in a high-risk group using color Doppler flow imaging in addition was confirmed by our group in 1993[14]. Twelve of 13 cardiac malformations could be diagnosed in 114 singleton pregnancies between 11 and 16 weeks of gestation. Only one case of an atrioventricular canal with double outlet right ventricle required a second-trimester transabdominal echocardiography at 20 weeks for the verification of the diagnosis. In several cases, however, additional malformations were overlooked, in particular anomalies of the great arteries, such as coarctation of the aorta[14].

To date, we have performed early echocardiography in 309 fetuses. In 78 of these cases, there were no known risk factors for cardiac malformation. In the remaining cases, the indications for echocardiography were fetal anomalies in 81 cases and anamnestic risk factors in 150. Cardiac malformations were diagnosed in 22 cases (7.1%) while the diagnosis was missed in four cases (1.3%) (Table 2). The latter included two cases with a ventricular defect detected at autopsy, an atrial septal defect of secundum type detected by postnatal echocardiography, and the above-mentioned case of atrioventricular canal and double outlet right ventricle. Atrioventricular valve regurgitation was demonstrated in six of these 22 cases.

The great majority of early diagnosed cardiac malformations in our series, as well as in the two series of Bronshtein and colleagues[21,22], were complex and severe. Amongst these were complete atrioventricular canal defect, single

**Table 2** Gestational age and diagnosis of 26 cases of congenital heart diseases by transvaginal two-dimensional and color Doppler echocardiography

| *Early diagnoses* | |
| --- | --- |
| 11 week | CAVC (1,2), CAVC, SV (1,2), SV, CoA |
| 12 week | CoA, large ASD II (1,2) |
| 13 week | CAVC |
| 14 week | CAVC, SV, HLH, VSD, VSD, TAC, dTGA + PA |
| 15 week | CAVC, DOLV + MA (1,2), VSD |
| 16 week | HLH, HLH, CoA, CoA |

| *Delayed and missed diagnoses* | |
| --- | --- |
| 12 weeks: 'normal' | 20 weeks: CAVC + DORV |
| 13 and 22 weeks: 'normal' | postpartum: ASD II |
| 12 weeks: early systolic | autopsy: VSD (trisomy 18) |
| 14 weeks: pansystolic | autopsy: VSD (trisomy 18) |

(1) Congenital heart disease with heterotaxia syndrome (four cases); (2) Congenital heart disease with atrioventricular block (four cases); ASD, atrial septal defect; CAVC, complete atrioventricular canal; CHD, congenital heart disease; CoA, coarctation of the aorta; DOLV, double outlet left ventricle; DORV, double outlet right ventricle; HLH, hypoplastic left heart; MA, mitral atresia; PA, pulmonary atresia; SV, single ventricle; dTGA, dextro-transposition of the great arteries; TR, tricuspid regurgitation; VSD, ventricular septal defect

ventricle, hypoplastic left heart (Color plates C–G), tubular coarctation of the aorta, large ventricular defect, tetralogy of Fallot, transposition of the great arteries and truncus arteriosus communis (Table 2). In some cases of atrioventricular canal defect, a heterotaxia (poly-splenia-/asplenia-) syndrome was also present.

## DIAGNOSIS OF ARRHYTHMIA

The observation of an atrioventricular block of second or third degree in the first or early second trimester seems to be nearly always associated with severe cardiac malformations, in particular heterotaxia syndromes. In our series of patients, a second-degree atrioventricular block diagnosed at 11 and 12 weeks' gestation and a third-degree atrioventricular block diagnosed at 11 and 15 weeks' gestation were associated with heterotaxia syndromes. It seems probable that a destruction of the fetal conducting system by maternal autoimmune antibodies of IgG type (anti-SSA- and anti-SSB-antibodies) generally occurs later in the gestation. A differentiation of arrhythmia in early pregnancy is possible using the same methods as in the second trimester. M-mode and/or pulsed wave Doppler echocardiography allow the measurement of the time interval between atrial and ventricular contractions by analyzing wall and valve movements and blood flow pattern. The MQ-mode, a combination of color-coded and M-mode Doppler echocardiography, allows simultaneous processing of conventional M-mode and Doppler echocardiography signals with a high time resolution. The analysis of intracardiac flow velocities as well as mechanical contraction and movement of valves allows conclusions to be drawn about electrical depolarization of the atria and ventricles, which in turn allows differentiation of the arrhythmia present. The earliest diagnosis of a supraventricular tachycardia was reported at 17 weeks' gestation[23].

## KARYOTYPING IN THE PRESENCE OF CARDIAC DEFECTS

The detection of a fetal cardiac malformation may be the first clue to the presence of a genetic syndrome or chromosomal abnormality. A comparison of karyotypes between a series of live births with cases of prenatally diagnosed congenital heart disease with a series of normal live births showed a 20–40% higher incidence of chromosomal defects in the former[24–26]. The high rate of spontaneous loss in early gestation suggests a higher rate of chromosomal anomalies in first-trimester fetuses with congenital heart disease. In our series of 26 fetuses with congenital heart diseases, 22 were diagnosed in early gestation and an abnormal karyotype was found in 15 of 26 fetuses (57%). On the other hand, our referral criteria for early echocardiography may cause an overrepresentation of chromosomal anomalies, e.g. due to the well-known association of nuchal edema with Down syndrome and of hygromata colli with Turner

syndrome (Figure 1). Nevertheless, rapid karyotyping by chorionic villi sampling seems to be mandatory once congenital heart disease is diagnosed. In the series of low-risk fetuses reported by Bronshtein and colleagues[22], 62% of those with early diagnosed cardiac defects showed extracardiac anomalies[22]. This may be explained by the high spontaneous loss rate of pregnancies with chromosomal abnormalities[25] as well as the disappearance of subtle anomalies[22] such as nuchal edema or mild dilatation of the renal pelvis.

## DISADVANTAGES AND PROBLEMS

There are some important disadvantages determining the diagnosis accuracy of transvaginal echocardiography when compared with a second-trimester examination. First, the imaging planes are limited by a narrow focal range, unfavorable fetal position or limited angles of insonation due to the more or less immobile transducer arc. Second, spatial orientation compared with transabdominal sonography is more difficult. This can lead to the presence of a visceral situs inversus or dextrocardia being overlooked. Therefore, a short transabdominal scan seems to be advisable since it is helpful in determining fetal orientation and the laterality of the stomach and heart[14]. Third, the most important limiting factor is the small size of the fetal heart, particularly before the 13th week of gestation. Small defects may escape diagnosis because of the limited resolution. This also applies to color Doppler flow imaging as the Doppler methods have a relatively low spatial resolution when compared with two-dimensional imaging. Low spatial resolution, lower frame rate, lower temporal resolution, and the small size of the inflow and outflow tract structures in the presence of a high heart rate make it difficult to obtain sharply divided blood flow patterns, particularly when a lower pulse repetition frequency is required.

Nevertheless, the biggest disadvantage of first-trimester echocardiography is the delayed progression of structural and functional cardiac changes in some forms of heart disease, thus manifesting themselves at a later gestational

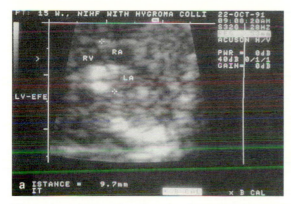

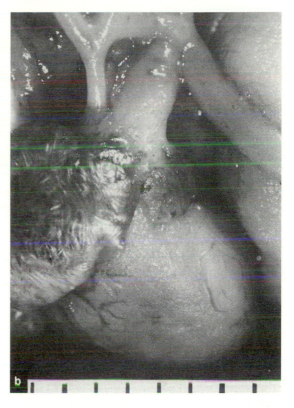

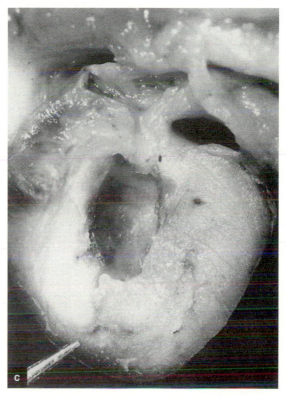

**Figure 1** (a) Four-chamber view in a case of Turner syndrome at 14 weeks + 5 days of gestation. The outer cardiac diameter at the level of the atrioventricular valves is marked by the two crosses. The lumen of the severely hypoplastic left ventricle was not visible and the whole left ventricular wall, including the interventricular septum, was hyperechogenic, indicating the presence of endocardial fibroelastosis (LA, left atrium; RA, right atrium; RV, right ventricle), as confirmed by autopsy; (b) stereomicroscopic picture of the fetal heart shows the severely hypoplastic ascending aorta, the relatively small aortic arch, the enlarged right atrial appendage and the broad pulmonary trunk and ductus arteriosus. The outside of the hypoplastic left ventricle is marked by the marginal branches of the anterior descending artery (on the right side); (c) stereomicroscopic picture shows the hypoplastic left ventricle and inflow tract and the very small posterior mitral leaflet. Reproduced with permission from Gembruch, U., Knöpfle, G., Bald, R. and Hansmann, M. (1993). Early diagnosis of fetal congenital heart disease by transvaginal echocardiography. *Ultrasound Obstet. Gynecol.*, **3**, 310–17

age. Myocardial hypertrophy, hypoplasia of one cardiac chamber and/or great artery in the presence of outflow tract obstructions (pulmonary stenosis, pulmonary atresia, aortic stenosis, aortic atresia, coarctation of the aorta) may be discernible only in the second or even in the third trimester[27–31]. This also seems to be true for the majority of cases with endocardial fibroelastosis. Therefore a diagnosis will not be able to be made by early two-dimensional echocardiography. It remains to be proven whether first-trimester diagnosis of severe stenosis or atresia of the pulmonary and aortic valve is possible using color Doppler flow imaging and pulsed wave Doppler. The presence of the turbulent or disturbed high-velocity jet of stenosis or reversed perfusion of the arterial trunk in question may point to the diagnosis. Dilatation of the atria secondary to atrioventricular-valve insufficiency (tricuspid valve dysplasia/Ebstein's anomaly, pulmonary atresia, atrioventricular canal defects) also seems to develop later in pregnancy and was rarely detected by early echocardiography. However, we were able successfully to demonstrate atrioventricular valve regurgitation in six cases using pulsed wave Doppler and color Doppler flow imaging in the first trimester.

## CONCLUSION

First-trimester fetal echocardiography should only be performed in high-risk fetuses between 13 and 15 weeks of gestation. The examination should predominantly be performed by transvaginal rather than transabdominal ultrasonography. Echocardiography in a low-risk group should be carried out between 18 and 20 weeks of gestation. We do not advocate routine screening of a low-risk group, as first-trimester echocardiography is less reliable than the second-trimester examination and thus may result in a higher false-positive and false-negative rate[14,22]. Even with the use of color-coded Doppler, additional cardiovascular anomalies accompanying the main cardiac defect may not be correctly diagnosed[14]. In some cases, these missed anomalies may be of considerable prognostic importance. In addition, the first-trimester examination is more time-consuming and requires a high level of training of the examiner. Furthermore, the examination is costly because of the required high-end equipment. Finally some cardiac lesions may not be detectable as the structural and functional progression of the lesion may only become apparent in the second or third trimester.

The high-risk group of patients to be scanned in the first trimester includes:

(1) Fetuses with other anomalies often occurring in association with cardiac defects, such as nuchal edema, hygroma colli, hydrops, omphalocele, situs inversus or persisting arrhythmia;

(2) High-risk families with one or more first-degree relatives with cardiac defects or those in which cardiac defects are either inherited by Mendelian rules alone, or as a part of a rare syndrome; and

(3) Fetuses with pregestational diabetes of the mother.

The examination should include and focus on the four-chamber view and visualization of the outflow tract using the segmental approach described below. If possible, color Doppler flow mapping should be used in addition. A follow-up examination by transabdominal echocardiography should always be performed in these high-risk patients because it markedly increases diagnostic accuracy and reliability. More detailed visualization of the larger cardiac structures during two-dimensional echocardiography and a better differentiation of intra- and extracardiac flow phenomena are the main advantages of second-trimester echocardiography.

For high-risk fetuses, early echocardiography should not be limited to the demonstration of the four-chamber view and the demonstration of the great arteries but is performed in a segmental approach[32]. We consider the use of color-coded Doppler as mandatory as it especially facilitates the demonstration of the veins and arteries and makes the visualization of intracardiac blood flow possible and thus is necessary for the detection of valvular insufficiencies. In the presence of complex malformation, diagnostic accuracy and speed of diagnosis are greatly enhanced. The position of the heart and its correlation to other intrathoracic and intra-abdominal organs must be documented first. Then, the inflow of the pulmonary veins into the left atrium and the venous inflow into the right atrium are demonstrated. Now the focus lies on the four-chamber view and the transition from the atria to the ventricles, the inflow tract with the atrioventricular valves. The next step is the visualization of the left and right ventricular outflow tract with the origin and crossing of the great arteries. Aortic arch and ductus arteriosus Botalli should also be visualized. Color Doppler flow imaging should make demonstration of the pulmonary venous inflow into the left atrium possible.

The diagnosis of cardiac malformations in the first trimester or even the exclusion of such defects is important, especially in families with a history of a child born with a hypoplastic left heart or similar lethal diseases, to reduce the severe anxiety of the parents early in pregnancy. With regard to the early development of cardiac malformations, the present data seem to be insufficient. Furthermore, normative growth charts must be confirmed by a larger number of patients. Pathological investigations after termination of pregnancy following the diagnosis of

a cardiac defect is of paramount importance to validate early echocardiography. When dilatation and curettage are performed for abortion, the conceptus is often severely damaged by the procedure, making a detailed and accurate pathological examination impossible. Therefore, we recommend induction of abortion using prostaglandin to allow for gentle extraction of the embryo, which is essential for a correct post-mortem diagnosis. Because of the small size of the specimen and the requirement for special examination techniques such as stereomicroscopy and high expertise of the examiner, we further recommend the pathological examination to be carried out in referral laboratories.

# References

1. Hoffman, J. I. E. (1990). Congenital heart disease: incidence and inheritance. *Pediatr. Clin. North. Am.*, **37**, 25–43
2. Allan, L. D., Anderson, R. H., Sullivan, I. D., Campbell, S., Holt, D. W. and Tynan, M. (1985). Spectrum of congenital heart disease detected echocardiographically in prenatal life. *Br. Heart J.*, **54**, 523–6
3. Gembruch, U., Chatterjee, M., Bald, R., Redel, D. A. and Hansmann, M. (1991). Color Doppler flow mapping of the fetal heart. *J. Perinat. Med.*, **19**, 27–32
4. Sharland, G. K., Chita, S. K. and Allan, L. D. (1990). The use of color Doppler in fetal echocardiography. *Int. J. Cardiol.*, **28**, 229–36
5. Allan, L. D. (1994). Fetal echocardiography (Editorial) *Ultrasound Obstet. Gynecol.*, **4**, 441–4
6. Achiron, R., Glasner, J., Gelernter, I., Hegesh, J. and Yagel, S. (1992). Extended fetal echocardiographic examination for detecting cardiac malformations in low risk pregnancies. *Br. Med. J.*, **304**, 671–4
7. Bromley, B., Estroff, J. A., Sanders, S. P., Parad, R., Roberts, D., Frigoletto, F. D. and Benacerraf, B. R. (1992). Fetal echocardiography: accuracy and limitations in a population at high and low risk for heart defects. *Am. J. Obstet. Gynecol.*, **166**, 1473–81
8. Sharland, G. K. and Allan, L. D. (1992). Screening for congenital heart disease prenatally. Results of a 2½-year study in the South East Thames Region. *Br. J. Obstet. Gynaecol.*, **99**, 220–5
9. Achiron, R. and Tadmor, O. (1991). Screening for fetal anomalies during the first trimester of pregnancy; transvaginal versus transabdominal sonography. *Ultrasound Obstet. Gynecol.*, **1**, 186–91
10. Cullen, M. T., Green, J., Whetham, J., Salafia, C., Gabrielli, S. and Hobbins, J. C. (1990). Transvaginal ultrasonographic detection of congenital anomalies in the first trimester. *Am. J. Obstet. Gynecol.*, **163**, 466–76
11. Rottem, S. and Bronshtein, M. (1990). Transvaginal sonographic diagnosis of congenital anomalies between 9 weeks and 16 weeks, menstrual age. *J. Clin. Ultrasound*, **18**, 307–14
12. Johnson, P., Sharland, G., Maxwell, D. and Allan, L. (1992). The role of transvaginal sonography in the early detection of congenital heart disease. *Ultrasound Obstet. Gynecol.*, **2**, 248–51
13. Dolkart, L. A. and Reimers, F. T. (1991). Transvaginal fetal echocardiography in early pregnancy: normative data. *Am. J. Obstet. Gynecol.*, **165**, 688–91
14. Gembruch, U., Knöpfle, G., Bald, R. and Hansmann, M. (1993). Early diagnosis of fetal congenital heart disease by transvaginal echocardiography. *Ultrasound Obstet. Gynecol.*, **3**, 310–17
15. Bronshtein, M., Siegler, E., Esheoli, Z. and Zimmer, E. Z. (1992). Transvaginal ultrasound

measurements of the fetal heart at 11 to 17 weeks of gestation. *Am. J. Perinatol.*, **9**, 38–42

16. Rizzo, G., Arduini, D. and Romanini, C. (1992). Doppler echocardiographic assessment of fetal cardiac function. *Ultrasound Obstet. Gynecol.*, **2**, 434–45

17. Wladimiroff, J. W., Stewart, P. A., Burghouwet, M. T. and Stijnen, T. (1992). Normal fetal cardiac flow velocity waveforms between 11 and 16 weeks of gestation. *Am. J. Obstet. Gynecol.*, **167**, 736–9

18. Huisman, T. W. A., Stewart, P. A. and Wladimiroff, J. W. (1992). Doppler assessment of the normal early fetal circulation. *Ultrasound Obstet. Gynecol.*, **2**, 300–5

19. Wladimiroff, J. W., Huisman, T. W. A., Stewart, P. A. and Stijnen, F. (1992). Normal fetal Doppler inferior vena cava, transtricuspid and umbilical artery flow velocity waveforms between 11 and 16 weeks' gestation. *Am. J. Obstet. Gynecol.*, **167**, 46–9

20. Gembruch, U., Knöpfle, G., Chatterjee, M., Bald, R. and Hansmann, M. (1990). First-trimester diagnosis of fetal congenital heart disease by transvaginal two-dimensional and Doppler echocardiography. *Obstet. Gynecol.*, **75**, 496–8

21. Bronshtein, M., Zimmer, E. Z., Milo, S., Ho, S. Y., Lorber, A. and Gerlis, L. M. (1991). Fetal cardiac abnormalities detected by transvaginal sonography at 12–16 weeks' gestation. *Obstet. Gynecol.*, **78**, 374–8

22. Bronshtein, M., Zimmer, E. Z., Gerlis, L. M., Lorber, A. and Drugan, A. (1993). Early ultrasound diagnosis of fetal congenital heart defects in high-risk and low-risk pregnancies. *Obstet. Gynecol.*, **82**, 225–9

23. Battiste, C. E., Neff, W., Evans, J. F. and Cline, B. W. (1992). *In utero* conversion of supraventricular tachycardia with digoxin and procainamide at 17 weeks' gestation. *Am. J. Perinatol.*, **9**, 302–3

24. Allan, L. D., Sharland, G. K., Chita, S. K., Lockhart, S. and Maxwell, D. J. (1991). Chromosomal anomalies in fetal congenital heart disease. *Ultrasound Obstet. Gynecol.*, **1**, 8–11

25. Berg, K. A., Clark, E. B., Astemborski, J. A. and Boughman, J. A. (1988). Prenatal detection of cardiovascular malformations by echocardiography: an indication for cytogenetic evaluation. *Am. J. Obstet. Gynecol.*, **69**, 494–7

26. Schwanitz, G., Zerres, K., Gembruch, U., Bald, R., Gamerdinger, F. and Hansmann, M. (1990). Prenatal detection of heart defects as an indication for chromosome analysis. *Ann. Génét.*, **33**, 79–83

27. Allan, L. D., Chita, S. K., Anderson, R. H., Fagg, N., Crawford, D. C. and Tynan, M. J. (1988). Coarctation of the aorta in prenatal life: an echocardiographic, anatomical, and functional study. *Br. Heart J.*, **59**, 356–60

28. Allan, L. D., Sharland, G. K. and Tynan, M. J. (1989). The natural history of the hypoplastic left heart syndrome. *Int. J. Cardiol.*, **25**, 341–3

29. Marasini, M., De Caro, E., Pongiglione, G., Ribaldone, D. and Caponnetto, S. (1993). Left heart obstructive disease with ventricular hypoplasia: changes in the echocardiographic appearance during pregnancy. *J. Clin. Ultrasound*, **21**, 65–8

30. Todros, T., Presbitero, P., Gaglioti, P. and Demarie, D. (1988). Pulmonary stenosis with intact ventricular septum: documentation of development of the lesion echocardiographically during fetal life. *Int. J. Cardiol.*, **19**, 355–60

31. Rice, M. J., McDonald, R. W. and Reller, M. D. (1993). Progressive pulmonary stenosis in the fetus: two case reports. *Am. J. Perinatol.*, **10**, 424–7

32. Huhta, J. C., Smallhorn, J. F. and McCartney, F. J. (1982). Two dimensional echocardiographic diagnosis of situs. *Br. Heart J.*, **48**, 97–103

# Prenatal diagnosis of congenital heart disease: septal defects and outflow obstructions

## 5

*P. Jeanty, D. Prandstraller, A. Perolo, G. Pilu, L. Bovicelli and F. M. Picchio*

## INTRODUCTION

Fetal echocardiography allows the antenatal diagnosis of congenital heart disease. The accuracy of this technique is nevertheless difficult to establish. Most antenatal series were obtained in populations at increased risk with an obvious bias towards the inclusion of prominent lesions of the fetal heart. The experience so far suggests that some anomalies are more likely to be detected than others. While the ascertainment of the connections between ventricles and great vessels requires meticulous scanning, a view of the four chambers of the heart can almost always be easily obtained. Anomalies involving the septa, and/or causing alterations in the size of the cardiac chambers represent the bulk of cases recognized antenatally.

In this chapter, we will discuss the principles for the antenatal diagnosis of these anomalies.

## ATRIAL SEPTAL DEFECTS

During embryogenesis, the common atrium is first divided by the septum primum into the right and left atria. The septum primum extends from the base of the heart towards the endocardial cushion. The gap between the two is called the ostium primum. When the fusion between the septum primum and the endocardial cushion has occurred, the septum primum fenestrates. The resulting communication between the two atria is called the ostium secundum. A second septum then extends on the right side of the septum primum and covers part of the ostium secundum. The remaining orifice is the foramen ovale, and the foramen ovale flap is the lower part of the septum primum. Thus, defects that are close to the endocardial cushion are called *ostium primum*, while defects in the area of the foramen ovale are *ostium secundum* defects. Ostium secundum defects are the most common, and are found in 0.07 per 1000 infants[1]. *Primum atrial septal defects* are the simplest form of the atrioventricular septal defects which will be considered later on.

*Secundum atrial septal defects* are most frequently isolated, but may be related to other cardiac lesions associated with interatrial shunts (such as mitral, pulmonary, tricuspid, or aortic atresia) and are occasionally found as part of syndromes, including Holt–Oram syndrome (ostium secundum defect, hypo-aplasia of the thumb and radius, triphalangeal thumb, abrachia, and phocomelia)[2].

Although the *in utero* identification of secundum atrial septal defect has been reported, the diagnosis remains difficult because of the physiological presence of the foramen ovale. Most likely, only unusually large defects can be recognized with certainty.

Atrial septal defects are not a cause of impairment of cardiac function *in utero*, as a large right-to-left shunt at the level of the atria is a physiological condition in the fetus. Most affected infants are asymptomatic even in the neonatal period.

## VENTRICULAR SEPTAL DEFECTS

Ventricular septal defects are probably the most common congenital cardiac defect, with an estimated incidence of 0.38 per 1000 live births[1]. They are classified into perimembranous, inlet, trabecular, or outlet defects depending on their location on the septum. *Perimembranous* defects (80%) are so called because they not only involve the membranous septum below the aortic valve, but extend to variable degrees into the adjacent portion of the septum. The *inlet* defects are on the inflow tract of the right ventricle and thus affect the implantation of the septal chordae of the tricuspid valve. The *trabecular* defects occur in the muscular portion of the septum, and the *outlet* defects are in the infundibular portion of the right ventricle. Trabecular defects (5–20%) have not been detected by prenatal ultrasound because they are usually composed of small orifices. Overall, small isolated ventricular septal defects are difficult to detect prenatally[3], and both false-positive and false-negative diagnoses have been made[4].

The echocardiographic diagnosis depends upon the demonstration of a dropout of echoes in the ventricular septum (Figure 1). While evaluating the ventricular septum in search of defects, multiple views should be used. Since most ventricular septal defects are perimembranous and subaortic, detailed views of the four chambers and of the left outflow tract are most helpful. Defects smaller than 1–2 mm will fall beyond the resolution power of current ultrasound equipment and will escape detection.

There is no evidence that ventricular septal defects are responsible for hemodynamic compromise *in utero*. Even a large interventricular communication gives rise probably only to small, bidirectional shunts in the fetus, as during intrauterine life the right and left ventricular pressures are believed to be equal[5]. It is debatable whether or not shunting across the defects can be detected by the use of color Doppler[6].

The vast majority of infants are not symptomatic in the neonatal period. Rare exceptions are represented by very large defects, associated with massive left-to-right shunt, that can indeed be associated with congestive heart failure soon after birth. Grossly, 25% of small trabecular defects close spontaneously, and a smaller proportion of the membranous defects also occlude.

## ATRIOVENTRICULAR SEPTAL DEFECTS

The ontogenesis of the apical portion of the atrial septum, of the basal portion of the interventricular septum and of the atrioventricular valves depends upon development of mesenchymal masses, defined as endocardial cushions. Abnormal development of these structures is commonly referred to as endocardial cushion defects, atrioventricular canal or atrioventricular septal defects. These anomalies are reported to occur in 0.12 per 1000 live births[1].

In the complete form, *persistent common atrioventricular canal*, the tricuspid and mitral valves are fused in a large scale atrioventricular valve that opens above and bridges the two ventricles. This valve has an anterior and a posterior leaflet. In the incomplete form, various amounts of tethering of one or both leaflets to the crest of the interventricular septum lead to connections that create functional atrial or ventricular septal defect, ventriculoatrial septal defect (connections between the left ventricle and right

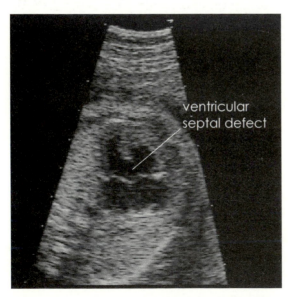

ventricular
septal defect

**Figure 1** Ventricular septal defect in a midtrimester fetus

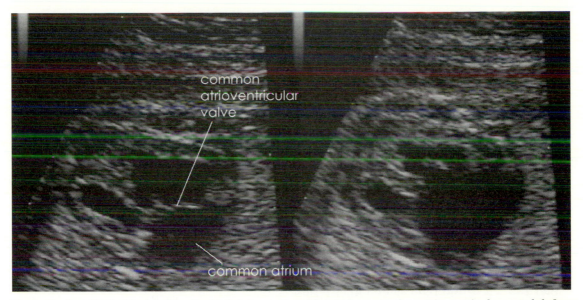

**Figure 2**  Systolic (left) and diastolic (right) frames in a fetus with a complete atrioventricular septal defect

atrium) or valvular abnormalities (clefting of the septal leaflet of the mitral valve).

In the complete form of atrioventricular canal, the common atrioventricular valve may be incompetent, and systolic blood regurgitation from the ventricles to the atria may give rise to congestive heart failure[7].

Antenatal echocardiographic diagnosis of complete atrioventricular septal defects is usually easy. An obvious deficiency of the central core structures of the heart is present (Figure 2). Color Doppler ultrasound can be useful, in that it facilitates the visualization of the central opening of the single atrioventricular valve (Color plate H). The atria may be dilated as a consequence of atrioventricular insufficiency. In such cases, color and pulsed Doppler ultrasound allow us to identify the regurgitant jet. The incomplete forms are more difficult to recognize. A useful hint is the demonstration that the tricuspid and mitral valves attach at the same level at the crest of the septum (Figure 3). This apical displacement of the mitral valve elongates the left ventricular outflow tract. The atrial septal defect is of the ostium primum type (since the septum secundum is not affected) and thus is close to the crest of the interventricular septum.

Atrioventricular septal defects will usually be encountered either in fetuses with chromoso-

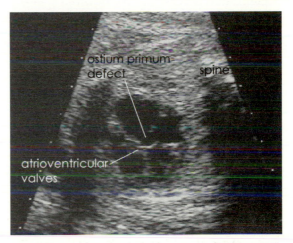

**Figure 3**  Ostium primum atrial septal defect. The four-chamber view demonstrates the absence of the septum primum; the atrioventricular valve insert is at the same level on the ventricular septum

mal aberrations (50% of cases are associated with aneuploidy, 60% being trisomy 21, 25% trisomy 18) or in fetuses with cardiosplenic syndromes[8]. In the former cases, an atrioventricular septal defect is frequently found in association with extracardiac anomalies. In the latter cases, multiple cardiac anomalies are almost the rule.

Non-cardiac anomalies include diaphragmatic hernia, duodenal atresia, omphalocele, lung agenesis, pleural effusions, hydrops, Melnick–Needles syndrome and cystic hygroma[9,10].

Atrioventricular septal defects do not impair fetal circulation *per se*. However, the presence of atrioventricular valve insufficiency may lead to intrauterine heart failure. The prognosis of atrioventricular septal defects is poor when detected *in utero*, probably because of the high frequency of associated anomalies in antenatal series. Only four out of 29 fetuses (14%) survived in one series, of which two had trisomy 21 and one was inoperable[8].

## CARDIOSPLENIC SYNDROMES

In cardiosplenic syndromes, the fetus is made of either two left or two right sides. Other terms commonly used include left or right isomerism, asplenia and polysplenia. As unpaired splanchnic organs (liver, stomach and spleen) may be absent, midline or duplicated, evaluation of the fetal abdominal organs is of special value for the sonographic diagnosis of these conditions.

In situs solitus and in situs inversus, the aorta and vena cava are on contralateral sides of the midline with the cava ipsilateral to the right atrium[11] (see Chapter 2). In polysplenia, the aorta is usually found on the midline, and the inferior vena cava is frequently interrupted. In asplenia, the aorta and cava are on the same side (either left or right) of the spine. In both conditions, the other abdominal organs often have an abnormal disposition (example, stomach to the right). Albeit the final diagnosis of the specific type of cardiac lesion is frequently a challenge even for the most experienced sonologists, in most cases the presence of the condition can be easily inferred from early gestation by a cross-section of the upper fetal abdomen.

### Polysplenia

Polysplenia is also defined as *left isomerism*, but it is not as distinctly 'double left-sided' as asplenia is 'double right-sided'. The stomach and aorta can be on opposite sides. The cardiac anomalies, although common, are less severe than those in asplenia. They include:

(1) Interrupted inferior vena cava with azygos continuation (75%);

(2) Partial anomalous pulmonary venous return (most commonly the pulmonary vein drains bilaterally to both atria);

(3) Bilateral superior venae cavae, each entering its own atrium;

(4) Rarely, transposition of the great arteries or double outlet right ventricle;

(5) Atrial septal defects, which tend to be smaller than those in asplenia;

(6) Obstructive lesions of the aortic valve; and

(7) Ventricular septal defect or atrioventricular septal defects.

In polysplenia, there are usually multiple spleens on both sides, that are, however, impossible to recognize with certainty with antenatal ultrasound. Although the spleen can be identified in normal fetuses[12], its absence is not a reliable finding[13] since the spleen can be difficult to visualize. The liver is most frequently found on the midline, and has symmetric lobes. In our experience, a symmetric liver can be sonographically recognized *in utero* by

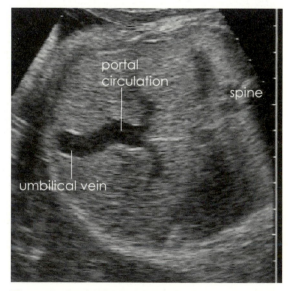

**Figure 4** In this fetus with polysplenia, the abnormal, symmetric disposition of the portal circulation suggests symmetry of the liver

demonstrating an abnormal course of the portal circulation, that does not display a clearly defined portal sinus bending to the right (Figure 4). Interruption of the inferior vena cava is also characteristic. In polysplenia, the cava is interrupted and continues into the hemiazygos, which is ipsilateral and posterior to the aorta. The azygos vein may drain to either superior vena cava; thus, the decussation of the azygos is not necessarily seen behind the bifurcation of the trachea. Finally, the hepatic vein does not join the inferior vena cava but crosses over to the left to empty in the azygos continuation or into the nearest atrium (not always the right atrium).

The most typical sonographic findings in fetal left isomerism include complex cardiac anomalies, abnormal disposition of the abdominal organs with a symmetric liver, failure to visualize the inferior vena cava entering the right atrium, and the presence of a large venous vessel, the azygos vein, running in the fetal chest posterior to the thoracic aorta (Figure 5)[14].

Associated anomalies include bilateral bilobated lungs, absence of the gallbladder and hypoplastic biliary structures, malrotation of the guts, duodenal atresia, preduodenal portal vein and hydrops. Left isomerism of the atria is frequently associated with absence of the sinus node, and this may lead in turn to bradycardia[10]. In most of the cases that we had an opportunity to follow throughout gestation, we have found that the baseline of the fetal cardiac frequency

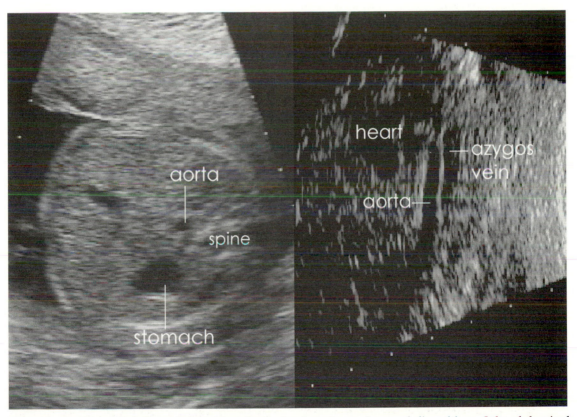

**Figure 5** In this midtrimester fetus with polysplenia, there is an abnormal disposition of the abdominal organs. In the left panel, a transverse cross-section of the upper abdomen fails to visualize the inferior vena cava, and demonstrates that the descending aorta is found in a central position. In the right panel, a sagittal view of the chest obtained from the back of the fetus is demonstrated. This view reveals a vessel, that had a venous pattern on pulsed Doppler, running posteriorly to the thoracic aorta. This identifies the vessel as an enlarged azygous vein, and suggests inferior vena cava interruption with azygous continuation

was between 90 and 110 beats per minute. Abnormalities of the atrioventricular junctions are also commonly found. Polysplenia is indeed one of the most frequent abnormalities associated with complete congenital atrioventricular block[15].

## Asplenia

In asplenia, or right isomerism, the fetus has two right sides. Thus, left side organs such as the spleen are rudimentary or absent. The liver is generally midline and the stomach right- or left-sided. The heart has two 'right atria'. The cardiac malformations are severe, with a tendency towards a single structure replacing normal paired structures: single atrium, single atrioventricular valve, single ventricle and single great vessel. The following are typically associated with asplenia:

(1) Bilateral superior vena cava;

(2) Double outlet right ventricle or pulmonary atresia;

(3) Large atrial septal defect (the interatrial septum is reduced to a fibrous band);

(4) Single atrioventricular valve and single ventricle;

(5) Total or partial anomalous pulmonary venous return (since there is no 'left' atrium, the pulmonary vein connects anomalously; the drainage is often either supracardiac or infradiaphragmatic, but, even when pulmonary veins enter the atrium, their morphology and connections are abnormal);

(6) Large ventricular septal defect;

(7) Transposition of the great arteries;

(8) Pulmonary restriction (stenosis or atresia).

The condition is more common in male fetuses, and few survive past the first few weeks or months. These newborns also suffer from a deficient immune system due to their asplenia. The diagnosis of asplenia can be confirmed in the newborn by doing a blood smear to detect the presence of Howell–Jolly and Heinz bodies. Al-

though we are unaware of this being performed on fetal blood, this seems simple enough to warrant trying it.

In asplenia, the cava is ipsilateral and anterior to the aorta, and the hepatic vein enters the atrium independently from the cava[16]. In the abdomen, the liver is transverse and the aorta and cava are on the same side (either left or right) of the spine. The spleen cannot be seen[13] and the stomach is found in close contact with the thoracic wall. The heterogeneous cardiac anomalies found in association with asplenia are usually easily seen, but a detailed diagnosis is usually a challenge. In particular, assessment of connection between the pulmonary veins and the atrium (an element that has a major prognostic influence) can be extremely difficult.

## AORTIC STENOSIS

Aortic stenosis, a condition that is found in 0.04 per 1000 live births[1], is commonly divided in supravalvar, valvar and subvalvar forms. Supravalvar aortic stenosis can be due to one of three anatomic defects: a membrane (usually placed above the sinuses of Valsalva), a localized narrowing of the ascending aorta (hour-glass deformity) or a diffuse narrowing involving the aortic arch and branching arteries (tubular variety). The valvar form of aortic stenosis, the most frequent one, can be due to dysplastic, thickened aortic cusps or fusion of the commissure between the cusps. The subvalvar forms include a fixed type, representing the consequence of a fibrous or fibromuscular obstruction, and a dynamic type, which is due to a thickened ventricular septum obstructing the outflow tract of the left ventricle. The former is usually an acquired lesion, that becomes evident only in postnatal life. The latter is also known as asymmetric septal hypertrophy or idiopathic hypertrophic subaortic stenosis[17]. A transient form of dynamic obstruction of the left outflow tract is seen in infants of diabetic mothers, and is probably the consequence of fetal hyperglycemia and hyperinsulinemia[18].

Echocardiographic diagnosis of valvar aortic stenosis depends upon real-time cross-sectional

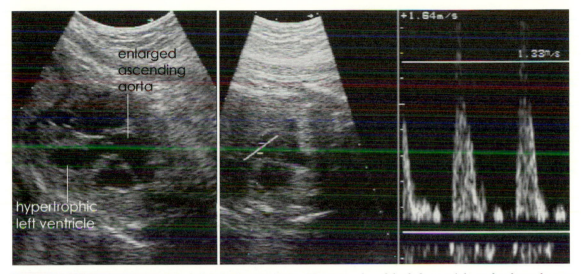

**Figure 6** Valvar aortic stenosis in a third-trimester fetus. Hypertrophy of the left ventricle and enlarged aorta with increased peak velocity of blood flow are demonstrated

demonstration of doming of the aortic cusps and Doppler ultrasound identification of post-stenotic turbulence (Figure 6). The increased work imposed upon the left ventricle leads to hypertrophy. Pulsed Doppler ultrasound is valuable for assessing both increased peak velocities in the ascending aorta, as well as insufficiency of the atrioventricular valves, that can accompany the cases with the most severe obstructions[19].

Asymmetric septal hypertrophy has been identified *in utero*[20]. The only reported case, however, is likely to be an exception, as there is evidence indicating that this anomaly has usually an evolutive course, and it is not apparent in the neonatal period[21]. An exception to this rule is represented by cases of secondary hypertrophic cardiomyopathies, such as those associated with maternal diabetes and congenital storage diseases. Prenatal diagnosis of hypertrophic cardiomyopathy in fetuses of diabetic mothers has been reported on several occasions[22]. We are not aware of cases of supravalvular aortic stenosis detected *in utero*.

In the most severe cases of aortic stenosis, the association of left ventricular pressure overload and subendocardial ischemia, due to decreased coronary perfusion, may lead to intrauterine impairment of cardiac function. Although subvalvular and subaortic forms are not generally manifested in the neonatal period, the valvar type can be a cause of congestive heart failure in the newborn and fetus as well[23]. Aortic stenosis is indeed one of the congenital cardiac defects most frequently found in association with intrauterine growth retardation[24].

Real-time and pulsed wave Doppler ultrasound allow a precise estimation of the severity of the stenosis. Knowledge of peak velocity allows the prediction of the pressure gradient with reasonable accuracy, by using the modified Bernoulli equation. There is concern that cases seen in early gestation may progress in severity. However, in the few cases we had an opportunity to follow throughout gestation, the lesions remained stable.

Aggressive management of fetal critical aortic stenosis with preterm delivery and early neonatal treatment has been advocated[25]. Invasive intrauterine treatment by balloon dilatation of the aortic valve has also been attempted, but the experience thus far is limited to a handful of cases[26].

## COARCTATION AND HYPOPLASTIC AORTIC ARCH

Coarctation is a localized narrowing of the juxtaductal arch, most commonly between the left subclavian artery and the ductus. It occurs in

0.18 per 1000 live births. A discrete shelf between the isthmus and the descending aorta is the most common finding at anatomic dissection. The pathogenesis of coarctation of the aorta is controversial. Three hypotheses have been suggested. Coarctation may be a true malformation, due to an embryogenetic abnormality, the consequence of aberrant ductal tissue in the aortic wall, resulting in narrowing of the isthmus at the time of closure of the ductus or, finally, the anatomic result of an intrauterine hemodynamic perturbance, due to an intracardiac anomaly diverting blood flow from the aorta into the pulmonary artery and the ductus arteriosus.

Hypoplastic aortic arch is a generalized narrowing of the aorta that affects the proximal arch, most commonly the segment between the left common carotid and the left subclavian artery or the isthmus, and may extend in the brachiocephalic vessels.

Cardiac anomalies are present in 90% of the cases and include aortic stenosis and insufficiency, ventricular septal defect, atrial septal defect, transposition of the great arteries, truncus and double outlet right ventricle.

The aortic valve is bicuspid in 25–50% of the cases. The mitral valve is abnormal in 25–50% of the cases[27]. Complete block may coexist[28].

Non-cardiac anomalies include, among the others, diaphragmatic hernia[29] and Turner syndrome.

Coarctation may be a postnatal event, and this limits prenatal diagnosis in many cases. However, this condition has been recognized in the fetus, albeit most frequently in late gestation[30,31]. An enlarged right ventricle (with a ratio over the left ventricle greater than 1.3) is usually found in these cases[31,32]. Most likely, the disproportion is secondary to an increase of blood flow in the ductus arteriosus to compensate the reduction in flow through the aortic isthmus. The index of suspicion increases when an echogenic shelf is found into the lumen of the aorta, or there is generalized narrowing (Figure 7)[31,32].

Albeit these findings do suggest the possible presence of coarctation, a certain diagnosis is difficult. We, as others, have found that, in many of these cases, the infants have no cardiac abnormalities whatsoever at birth. On the other hand,

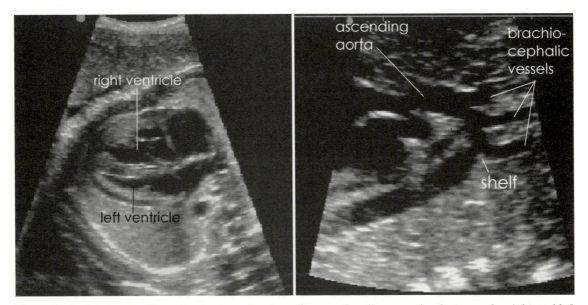

**Figure 7** In this fetus at 32 weeks, the four-chamber view reveals a disproportion between the right and left ventricles. A sagittal view of the aortic arch suggests the presence of a shelf distal to the brachiocephalic vessels. A previous echocardiogram had been performed in the midtrimester and was unremarkable. Coarctation of the aorta was confirmed after birth

coarctation may be found in cases with an unremarkable antenatal echocardiogram[33,34].

As the blood flow through the isthmus is minimal during intrauterine life, the descending aorta being mainly supplied via the ductus arteriosus, isolated coarctation is not expected to alter significantly the hemodynamics. However, cases with hypoplastic aortic arch may result in a greater hemodynamic burden.

## INTERRUPTED AORTIC ARCH

The interruption can be complete or there may be an atretic fibrous segment between the arch and the descending aorta. The lesion has been considered an extreme form of coarctation[35]. The interruptions are categorized according to their level compared to the brachiocephalic vessels. In type A (42%), the aorta supplies the three brachiocephalic vessels, and the pulmonary artery supplies the descending aorta via the ductus[36]. In type B (53%), the interruption is proximal to the left subclavian artery. In type C (4%), the interruption is between the right innominate and left common carotid artery. Type C is the most lethal form. A common anomaly (which is still probably beyond prenatal recognition) is the presence of a replaced right subclavian artery that originates from the distal portion of the aorta. Ventricular septal defects are almost always present in type B and occur in 50% of type A.

Associated cardiac anomalies include atrial septal defect, subaortic stenosis, hypoplasia of the ascending aorta, bicuspid aortic and/or pulmonic valve, replaced right subclavian artery and ventricular septal defects. The ventricular septal defect is of the malalignment type with obstruction of the aortic outflow.

Associated extracardiac anomalies include DiGeorge syndrome (thymic aplasia, type B interruption and hypoplastic mandible), holoprosencephaly, cleft lip/palate, esophageal atresia, duplicated stomach, diaphragmatic hernia, horseshoe kidneys, bilateral renal agenesis, oligodactyly, claw hand and syrenomelia.

The characteristic findings of an *arch* in the higher chest from which no or too few vessels originate should suggest the diagnosis[37,38]. In a sagittal section, the aorta can be traced into the carotids but cannot be traced into the descending aorta (Figure 8). Another finding is the discrepancy between the size of the aorta and the pulmonary artery, which is larger.

Interrupted aortic arch is not supposed to cause *in utero* heart failure *per se*. However, the hemodynamics largely depend upon the associated cardiac malformations. The prognosis is severe for untreated infants, with a median age at death of 4 days[39].

## HYPOPLASTIC LEFT HEART

Hypoplastic left heart syndrome is characterized by a very small left ventricle, with mitral and/or aortic atresia. Blood flow to the head and neck vessels and coronary artery is supplied in a retrograde manner via the ductus arteriosus. This condition has been described in 0.16 per 1000 live births[1].

Echocardiographic diagnosis of hypoplastic left heart syndrome in the fetus depends upon the demonstration of a diminutive left ventricle and ascending aorta[40,41]. In most cases, the ultrasound appearance is self-explanatory, and the diagnosis an easy one (Figure 9). There is,

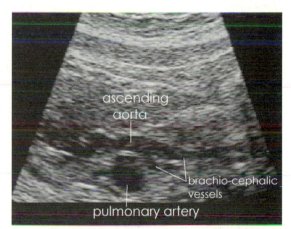

**Figure 8** In this third-trimester fetus with mitral atresia, the ascending aorta is smaller than usual, and relative to the large pulmonary artery as well. The course of the vessel is more vertical than normal, and it was impossible to demonstrate a connection with the descending aorta. Interruption of the aortic arch was confirmed after birth

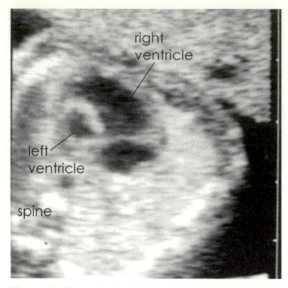

**Figure 9** Hypoplastic left heart syndrome in a 22-week fetus. The echogenic internal lining of the small ventricle is probably due to an associated endocardial fibroelastosis. On real-time examination, the ventricular walls did not show any contractility, and the mitral valve did not open

however, a broad spectrum of hypoplasia of the left ventricle. We have seen cases with a ventricular cavity of almost normal size, that may indeed represent a diagnostic challenge, particularly in early gestation. The definitive diagnosis of hypoplastic left heart syndrome depends, however, upon demonstration of hypoplasia of the ascending aorta and atresia of the aortic valve. Color flow imaging is an extremely useful adjunct to the real-time examination, in that it allows the demonstration of retrograde blood flow within the ascending aorta and aortic arch (Color plate I).

The prognosis for untreated infants with hypoplastic left heart syndrome is extremely poor. This lesion is responsible for 25% of cardiac deaths in the first week of life[42]. In the last decade, Norwood's three-stage operation as the elective corrective procedure has undergone great diffusion in many countries. It is presently acknowledged that, albeit the surgical risk is 30–40%, the midterm prognosis for operated infants is good. Long-term prognosis remains uncertain[43]. Recently, cardiac transplantation

in the neonatal period has also been attempted[44].

Hypoplastic left heart is well tolerated *in utero*. The patency of the ductus arteriosus allows adequate perfusion of the head and neck vessels. Intrauterine growth may be normal, and the onset of symptoms most frequently occurs after birth. Congestive heart failure is only seen in cases with insufficiency of the atrioventricular valves; these, however, represent a distinct minority.

## PULMONARY STENOSIS

The most common form of pulmonary stenosis is the valvar type, due to the fusion of the pulmonary leaflets. Hemodynamics are altered proportionally to the degree of the stenosis. The work of the right ventricle is increased, as well as the pressure, leading to hypertrophy of the ventricular walls. In the most severe cases, that represent, however, rare exceptions, right ventricular overload may result in congestive heart failure.

The same considerations formulated for the prenatal diagnosis of aortic stenosis are valid for pulmonic stenosis as well. A handful of cases recognized *in utero* have been reported in the literature thus far, mostly severe types with enlargement of the right ventricle and/or poststenotic enlargement or hypoplasia of the pulmonary artery. Intrauterine development, with an unremarkable midtrimester echocardiogram, has also been documented[45].

## PULMONARY ATRESIA WITH INTACT VENTRICULAR SEPTUM

Pulmonary atresia with intact ventricular septum in infants is usually associated with a hypoplastic right ventricle. However, cases with enlarged right ventricle and atrium have been described with unusual frequency in prenatal series[46]. Although prenatal series are small, it is possible that the discrepancy with the pediatric literature is due to the very high perinatal loss rate that is found in 'dilated' cases. Enlargement of the ventricle and atrium is the consequence of tricuspid insufficiency. Prenatal diagnosis of pulmonary atresia with intact ventricular septum relies upon the demonstration of a small pulmonary artery with an atretic pulmonary valve. Color/pulsed Doppler are both valuable for assessing both retrograde blood flow within the pulmonary artery as well as the presence of tricuspid insufficiency in 'dilated' cases (Color plate J).

In cases with tricuspid insufficiency, intrauterine heart failure and hydrops may develop. On the other hand, in the absence of tricuspid regurgitation, pulmonary atresia is well tolerated, and the onset of symptoms only occurs after birth.

## UNIVENTRICULAR HEART

The term 'univentricular heart' defines a group of anomalies characterized by the presence of an atrioventricular junction that is entirely connected to only one chamber in the ventricular mass. The univentricular heart includes, therefore, both those cases in which the two atrial chambers are connected, by either two distinct atrioventricular valves or by a common one, to a main ventricular chamber (classic double-inlet single ventricle), as well as those cases in which, because of the absence of one atrioventricular connection (tricuspid or mitral atresia), one of the ventricular chambers is either rudimentary or absent. The main ventricular chamber may be either the left or right type, and in some cases may be of indeterminate type. A rudimentary ventricular chamber lacking atrioventricular connection is a frequent but not constant finding. The double inlet left ventricle is the most frequent form, accounting for more than 70% of all forms. Ventriculo-arterial connections can be either concordant or discordant, depending on the connection of the great arteries to the main ventricular chamber. Single or double outlet can occur from the main chamber as well as from the rudimentary ventricle.

Antenatal echocardiographic diagnosis is usually easy (Figure 10). The presence of a single ventricle is not a cause of heart failure *per se*. However, the hemodynamics may vary greatly from case to case, depending upon the type of ventriculo-arterial connection and the sum of the associated cardiac anomalies that are very frequently seen.

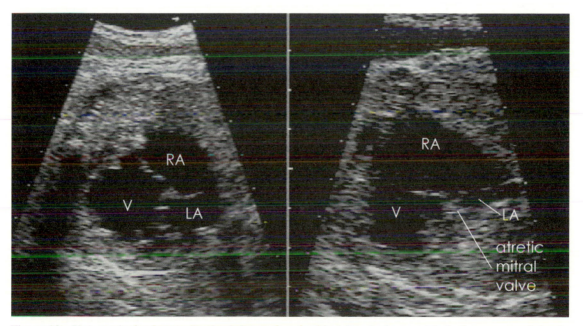

**Figure 10** Univentricular hearts. In the left panel, a double inlet single ventricle is demonstrated; in the right panel, mitral atresia is shown. (RA, LA indicate the right and left atria, V, the single ventricular cavity)

# References

1. Fyler, D. C., Buckley, L. P., Hellenbrand, W. E., Cohn, H. E., Kirklin, J. W., Nadas, A. S., Cartier, J. M. and Breibart, M. H. (1980). Report of the New England Regional Cardiac Program. *Pediatrics*, **65** (Suppl.), 375–461

2. Brons, J. T., van Geijn, H. P., Wladimiroff, J. W., van Der Harten, J. J., Kwee, M. L., Sobotka-Plojhar, M. and Arts, N. F. (1988). Prenatal ultrasound diagnosis of the Holt Oram syndrome. *Prenat. Diagn.*, **8**, 175–81

3. Benacerraf, B. R., Pober, B. R. and Sanders, S. P. (1987). Accuracy of fetal echocardiography. *Radiology*, **165**, 847–9

4. Marasini, M., Cordone, M., Pongiglione, G., Lituania, M., Bertolini, A. and Ribladone, D. (1988). *In utero* ultrasound diagnosis of congenital heart disease. *J. Clin. Ultrasound*, **16**, 103–7

5. Rudolph, A. M. (1974). *Congenital Disease of the Heart*. (Chicago: Year Book Medical Publisher)

6. Gembruch, U., Hansmann, M., Redel, D. A. and Bald, R. (1988). 2-dimensional color-coded fetal Doppler echocardiography – its value in prenatal diagnosis. *Geburtshilfe Frauenheilkd.*, **48**, 381–8

7. Kleinman, C. S., Donnerstein, R. L., DeVore, G. R., Jaffe, C. C., Lynch, D. C., Berkowitz, R. L., Talner, N. S. and Hobbins, J. C. (1982). Fetal echocardiography for evaluation of *in utero* congestive heart failure: a technique for study of nonimmune fetal hydrops. *N. Engl. J. Med.*, **306**, 568–75

8. Machado, M. V., Crawford, D. C., Anderson, R. H. and Allan, L. D. (1988). Atrioventricular septal defect in prenatal life. *Br. Heart J.*, **59**, 352–5

9. Donnenfeld, A. E., Conard, K. A., Roberts, N. S., Borns, P. F. and Zackai, E. H. (1987). Melnick–Needles syndrome in males: a lethal multiple congenital anomalies syndrome. *Am. J. Med. Genet.*, **27**, 159–73

10. Gembruch, U., Hansmann, M., Redel, D. *et al.* (1988). Non immunologically induced hydrops fetalis in complete atrioventricular block of the fetus. A summary of 11 prenatally diagnosed cases. *Geburtshilfe Frauenheilkd.*, **48**, 494–9

11. Huhta, J. C., Smallhorn, J. F. and Macartney, F. J. (1982). Cross-sectional echocardiographic diagnosis of situs. *Br. Heart J.*, **48**, 97–108

12. Schmidt, W., Yarkoni, S., Jeanty, P., Reece, E. A. and Hobbins, J. C. (1985). Sonographic measurements of the fetal spleen: clinical implications. *J. Ultrasound Med.*, **4**, 667–72

13. Chitayat, D., Lao, A., Wilson, R. D., Fagerstrom, C. and Hayden, M. (1988). Prenatal diagnosis of asplenia/polysplenia syndrome. *Am. J. Obstet. Gynecol.*, **158**, 1085–7

14. Sheley, R. C., Nyberg, D. A. and Kapur, R. (1995). Azygous continuation of the interrupted inferior vena cava: a clue to prenatal diagnosis of cardiosplenic syndromes. *J. Ultrasound Med.*, **14**, 381–7

15. Schmidt, K. G., Ulmer, H. E., Silverman, N. H., Kleinman, C. S. and Copel, J. A. (1991). Perinatal outcome of fetal complete atrioventricular block: a multicenter experience. *J. Am. Coll. Cardiol.*, **17**, 1360–6

16. Stewart, P. A., Becker, A. E., Wladimiroff, J. W. and Essed, C. E. (1984). Left atrial isomerism associated with asplenia: prenatal echocardiographic detection of complex congenital cardiac malformations. *J. Am. Coll. Cardiol.*, **4**, 1015–20

17. Becker, A. E. and Anderson, R. H. (1981). *Pathology of Congenital Heart Disease*. (London: Butterworths)

18. Walther, F. J., Siassi, B. and King, J. (1985). Cardiac output in infants of insulin-dependent diabetic mothers. *J. Pediatr.*, **107**, 109–14

19. Kenny, J. F., Plappert, T., Doubilet, P., Salzman, D. and Sutton, M. G. (1987). Effects of heart rate on ventricular size, stroke, volume, and output in the normal human fetus: a prospective Doppler echocardiographic study. *Circulation*, **76**, 52–8

20. Stewart, P. A., Buis-Liem, T., Verwey, R A. and Wladimiroff, J. W. (1986). Prenatal ultrasonic diagnosis of familial asymmetric septal hypertrophy. *Prenat. Diagn.*, **6**, 249–56

21. Wright, G. B., Keane, J. F. and Nadas, A. S. (1983). Fixed subaortic stenosis in the young. Medical and surgical course in 83 patients. *Am. J. Cardiol.*, **52**, 830–7

22. Rizzo, G., Arduni, D. and Romanini, C. (1992). Accelerated cardiac growth and abnormal cardiac flows in fetuses of type I diabetic mothers. *Obstet. Gynecol.*, **80**, 369–76

23. Allan, L. D., Little, D., Campbell, S. and Whitehead, M. I. (1981). Fetal ascites associated with congenital heart disease. Case report. *Br. J. Obstet. Gynaecol.*, **88**, 453–5

24. Reynolds, J. L. (1972). Intrauterine growth retardation in children with congenital heart disease. Its relation to aortic stenosis. *Birth Defects Original Articles Series*, **8**, 143–57

25. Huhta, J. C., Carpenter, R. J., Moise, K. J. Jr, Deter, R. L., Ott, D. A. and McNamara, D. G. (1987). Prenatal diagnosis and postnatal management of critical aortic stenosis. *Circulation*, **75**, 573–6

26. Maxwell, D., Allan, L. D. and Tynan, M. J. (1991). Balloon dilatation of the aortic valve in the fetus: a report of two cases. *Br. Heart J.*, **65**, 256–8

27. Becker, A. E., Becker, M. J. and Edwards, J. E. (1970). Anomalies associated with coarctation of the aorta. *Circulation*, **41**, 1067–72

28. Machado, M. V., Tynan, M. J., Curry, P. V. and Allan, L. D. (1988). Fetal complete heart block. *Br. Heart J.*, **60**, 512–15

29. Siebert, J. R., Hass, J. E. and Beckwith, J. B. (1984). Left ventricular hypoplasia in congenital diaphragmatic hernia. *J. Pediatr. Surg.*, **19**, 567–71

30. Allan, L. D., Crawford, D. C. and Tynan, M. J. (1984). Evolution of coarctation of the aorta in intrauterine life. *Br. Heart J.*, **52**, 471–4

31. Allan, L. D., Chita, S. K., Anderson, R. H., Fagg, N., Crawford, D. C. and Tynan, M. J. (1988). Coarctation of the aorta in prenatal life: an echocardiographic, anatomical, and functional study. *Br. Heart J.*, **59**, 356–60

32. Benacerraf, B. R., Saltzman, D. H. and Sanders, S. P. (1989). Sonographic sign suggesting the prenatal diagnosis of coarctation of the aorta. *J. Ultrasound Med.*, **8**, 65–9

33. Sharland, G. K., Chan, K. Y. and Allan, L. D. (1994). Coarctation of the aorta. Difficulties in prenatal diagnosis. *Br. Heart J.*, **71**, 70–5

34. Hornberg, L. K., Sahn, D. J., Kleinman, C. S., Copel, J. and Silverman, N. H. (1994). Antenatal diagnosis of coarctation of the aorta: a multicenter experience. *J. Am. Coll. Cardiol.*, **23**, 417–23

35. Van Mierop, L. and Kutsche, L. M. (1971). Interruption of the aortic arch and coarctation of the aorta: pathogenetic relations. *Am. J. Cardiol.*, **54**, 829–37

36. Celoria, G. C. and Patton, R. B., (1959). Congenital absence of the aortic arch. *Am. Heart J.*, **58**, 407–13

37. Marasini, M., Cordone, M., Zampatti, C., Pongiglione, G., Bertolini, A. and Ribaldone, D. (1987). Prenatal ultrasonic detection of truncus arteriosus with interrupted aortic arch and truncal valve regurgitation. *Eur. Heart J.*, **8**, 921–4

38. Johnson, B. L., Fyfe, D. A., Gillette, P. C., Kline, C. H. and Sade, R. (1989). *In utero* diagnosis of interrupted aortic arch with transposition of the great arteries and tricuspid atresia. *Am. Heart J.*, **117**, 690–2

39. Collins-Nakia, R., Dick, M. and Parisi-Buckley, L. (1976). Interrupted aortic arch in infancy. *J. Pediatr.*, **88**, 959–62

40. Sahn, D. J., Shenker, L., Reed, K. L., Valdes-Cruz, L. M., Sobonya, R. and Anderson, C. (1982). Prenatal ultrasound diagnosis of hypoplastic left heart syndrome *in utero* associated with hydrops fetalis. *Am. Heart J.*, **104**, 1368–72

41. Silverman, N. H., Enderlein, M. A. and Golbus, M. S. (1984). Ultrasonic recognition of aortic valve atresia *in utero*. *Am. J. Cardiol.*, **53**, 391

42. Doty, D. B. (1980). Aortic atresia. *J. Thorac. Cardiovasc. Surg.*, **79**, 462

43. Jonas, R. A., Hansen, D. D., Cook, N. and Wessel, D. (1994). Anatomic subtype and survival after reconstructive operation for hypoplastic left heart syndrome. *J. Thorac. Cardiovasc. Surg.*, **107**, 1121–8

44. Bailey, L. L., Gundry, S. R., Razzouk, A. J., Wang, N., Sciolaro, C. M., Chiavarelli, M. and the Loma Linda University Pediatric Heart Transplant Group (1993). Bless the babies: one hundred fifteen late survivors of heart transplantation during the first year of life. *J. Thorac. Cardiovasc. Surg.*, **105**, 805–15

45. Todros, T., Presbitero, P., Gagliotti, J. and Demarie, D. (1988). Pulmonary stenosis with intact ventricular septum: documenation of the development of the lesion echocardiographically during fetal life. *Int. J. Cardiol.*, **19**, 355–60

46. Allan, L. D., Crawford, D. C. and Tynan, M. J. (1986). Pulmonary atresia in prenatal life. *J. Am. Coll. Cardiol.*, **8**, 1131–5

# Prenatal diagnosis of conotruncal malformations

6

*D. Prandstraller, G. Pilu, A. Perolo, F. M. Picchio and L. Bovicelli*

## INTRODUCTION

Conotruncal malformations are a heterogeneous group of defects that involve two different segments of the heart: the conotruncus and the ventricles. They include: transposition of the great arteries, double outlet right ventricle, tetralogy of Fallot, pulmonary atresia with ventricular septal defect and truncus arteriosus communis.

Conotruncal anomalies are relatively frequent. They account for 20–30% of all cardiac anomalies[1] and are the leading cause of symptomatic cyanotic heart disease in the first year of life. Prenatal diagnosis is of interest for several reasons. Given the parallel model of fetal circulation, conotruncal anomalies are well tolerated *in utero*. The clinical presentation occurs usually hours to days after delivery, and is often severe, representing a true emergency and leading to considerable morbidity and mortality. Yet, these malformations have a good prognosis when promptly treated. Two ventricles of adequate size and two great vessels are commonly present giving the premise for biventricular surgical correction. The outcome is indeed much more favorable than with most of the other cardiac defects that are detected antenatally.

The first reports on prenatal echocardiography of conotruncal malformations date back from the beginning of the 1980s[2–4]. Nevertheless, despite improvement in the technology of diagnostic ultrasound, the recognition of these anomalies remains difficult. The four-chamber view, that many recommend to include in the standard sonographic examination of fetal anatomy, is frequently unremarkable in these cases[5]. A specific diagnosis requires meticulous scanning and at times may represent a challenge even for experienced sonologists. Referral centers with special expertise in fetal echocardiography have indeed reported both false-positive[4] and false-negative[6] diagnoses.

In this chapter, the main diagnostic and clinical features of conotruncal anomalies will be reviewed, with special emphasis on the issue of antenatal identification.

## APPROACH TO ANTENATAL ECHOCARDIOGRAPHIC DIAGNOSIS

Echocardiographic diagnosis of conotruncal anomalies requires accurate assessment of ventriculo-arterial connections. The antenatal approach is similar to the one described for neonates[7]. In the normal fetal heart, long-axis views of the ventricles allow adequate visualization of the outflow tracts and origin of the great arteries. An important clue to the diagnosis of many conotruncal anomalies is the sonographic demonstration of the relation between the great vessels, that cross under normal conditions. This can be demonstrated by either sequential visualization of each outflow tract or by simultaneous demonstration of both vessels in a short-axis view. The vessels can then be identified by following their course to the aortic arch and pulmonary bifurcation (Figure 1).

When adequate resolution can be achieved and the fetus is in a favorable position, the ventriculo-arterial connections can be rapidly and easily assessed around mid-gestation with standard transabdominal sonography[8], and in most cases from 12–13 weeks by using high-frequency transvaginal probes[9].

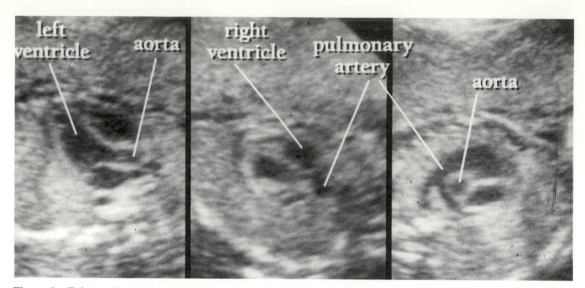

**Figure 1** Echocardiographic demonstration of normal ventriculo-arterial connections in a midtrimester fetus. Images are oriented with left side of the fetus to the left. In the left panel, the connection between the left ventricle and the ascending aorta is demonstrated by a long-axis view. Note mitro-aortic continuity, and the upward course of the aorta. The central panel shows a long-axis view of the right ventricle, demonstrating the outflow tract of the right ventricle and the pulmonary artery that has a posterior course, crossing over the aorta. In the right panel, a short-axis view of the great vessels is demonstrated, with the right atrium, outflow tract of right ventricle, and pulmonary artery wrapping around a cross-section of the ascending aorta. The bifurcation of the main pulmonary artery is also seen

However, in a fetus that is actively moving, or keeping unfavorable positions, it may be time-consuming and frustrating to obtain proper views, particularly when an anomaly is present and the normal anatomic relationships are altered. Indeed, assessment of ventriculo-arterial connections is commonly regarded as the most difficult part of the fetal echocardiographic examination. Similarly to others[10] we have found color Doppler useful, in that it allows accurate demonstration of the outflow tracts in many situations in which the visualization with gray-scale bidimensional ultrasound is suboptimal because of inadequate angling or poor resolution.

Echocardiographic evaluation of conotruncal anomalies requires multiple plane imaging to demonstrate the following:

(1) Complete sequential approach in order to define situs, position of the heart in the thorax, venous returns, atrioventricular and ventriculo-arterial connections;

(2) Four-chamber view to assess ventricular size and function;

(3) Transverse (short-axis) view of the great vessels, to assess topographic relation and relative size of the vessels;

(4) Long-axis views of the ventricles (equivalent of the classic subcostal views, both left and right oblique traditionally employed in postnatal echocardiography) to assess outflow tracts and connections;

(5) Morphology of the arch and functional assessment of ductus arteriosus direction of flow;

(6) Morphology of atrioventricular valves and identification of straddling or of other major abnormality, as far as possible, from prenatal views;

(7) Pulsed wave Doppler and color coding are eventually important in many cases to demonstrate presence, direction and characteristics of blood flow across the valves.

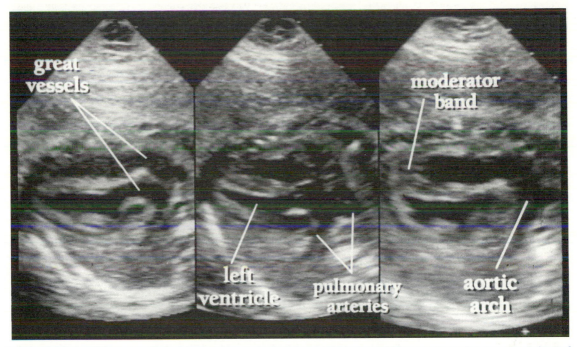

**Figure 2** Complete transposition of the great vessels, simple form, in a 31-week fetus. Images are oriented with the left side of the fetus to the left. Left panel, contrarily to normal, in a long-axis view of the heart the two great vessels are seen simultaneously, and appear to arise parallel from the base of the heart. This attests an abnormal relationship between the great vessels that is in itself diagnostic of transposition. Central panel, the posterior ventricle is morphologically of the left type (no moderator band at the apex, continuity between the atrioventricular and the semilunar valve) and in a long-axis view appears to be connected with a great vessel that has a posterior course and bifurcates, thus identifying itself as the pulmonary artery. Right panel, the anterior ventricle is morphologically of the right type (presence of the moderator band at the apex, discontinuity between atrioventricular and semilunar valve) but is connected with a vessel that can be positively identified as the aorta by its long upward course and by the connection with brachiocephalic vessels

## TRANSPOSITION OF THE GREAT ARTERIES

Transposition of the great arteries (TGA) is most commonly found in the complete form, which is characterized by atrioventricular concordance with ventriculo-arterial discordance. The aorta arises from the right ventricle and lies anterior and leftward to the pulmonary artery, that is connected to the left ventricle and lies posterior and medial. The most common form is the setting of the so-called dextro-TGA.

The prevalence is two per 10 000 live births[1]. Associated lesions are present in roughly 50% of cases, including ventricular septal defects (which can occur anywhere in the ventricular septum), pulmonary stenosis, unbalanced ventricular size ('complex transpositions'), and anomalies of the mitral valve, which can be straddling or overriding.

According to Becker and Anderson[11], three types of complete TGA can be distinguished: TGA with intact ventricular septum with or without pulmonary stenosis; TGA with ventricular septal defects; and TGA with ventricular septal defects and pulmonary stenosis.

Complete transposition is probably one of the most difficult cardiac lesions to recognize *in utero*. In most cases, the four-chamber view is normal, and the cardiac cavities and the vessels are normal. A clue to the diagnosis is the demonstration that the two great vessels do not cross but arise parallel from the base of the heart (Figure 2). The most useful echocardiographic

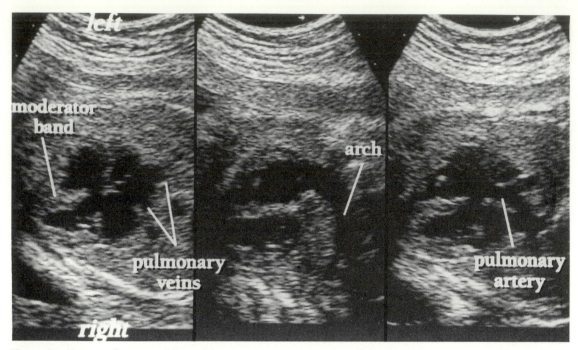

**Figure 3** Corrected transposition of the great arteries in a 33-week fetus. Images are oriented with the left side of the fetus upward. Left panel, apart from obvious dextrocardia, a four-chamber view reveals findings that are by themselves diagnostic of atrioventricular discordance: there is a perimembranous ventricular septal defect, the posterior ventricle is morphologically of the right type (the moderator band is seen at the apex) and is connected with an atrium in which the pulmonary veins enter. Central panel, a long-axis view of the posterior, morphologically right ventricle, demonstrates that this is connected with a vessel that has a long upward course and that can therefore be identified as the ascending aorta. Right panel, a small pulmonary artery is seen overriding the ventricular septal defect. Pulsed wave ultrasound attested increased peak velocities into this vessel, corroborating the diagnosis of pulmonic stenosis

view *in utero* is, however, the equivalent of the subcostal oblique in postnatal life[7] demonstrating that the vessel connected to the left ventricle has a posterior course and bifurcates into the two pulmonary arteries. Conversely, the vessel connected to the right ventricle has a long upward course and gives rise to the brachiocephalic vessels.

Difficulties may arise in the case of huge malalignment ventricular septal defects with overriding of the posterior semilunar root. This combination makes the differentiation from double outlet right ventricle very difficult.

Corrected TGA is characterized by a double discordance, at the atrioventricular and ventriculo-arterial levels. The left atrium is connected to the right ventricle, which is in turn connected to the ascending aorta. Conversely, the right atrium is connected with the right ventricle, which is in turn connected to the ascending aorta. The derangement of the conduction tissue secondary to malalignment of the atrial and ventricular septa may result in dysrhythmias, namely complete atrioventricular block[12].

For diagnostic purposes, the identification of the peculiar difference of ventricular morphology (moderator band, papillary muscles, insertion of the atrioventricular valves) has a pre-eminent role. Demonstration that the pulmonary veins are connected to an atrium which is in turn connected with a ventricle that has the moderator band at the apex is an important clue, that is furthermore potentially identifiable even in a simple four-chamber view (Figure 3). Diagnosis requires meticulous scanning to assess carefully all cardiac connections, by using the same views described for the complete form.

The presence of atrioventricular block increases the index of suspicion[12].

As anticipated from the parallel model of fetal circulation, complete TGA is uneventful *in utero*. The lack of hemodynamic compromise is indirectly attested by the frequency of a normal birth weight in these infants. After birth, survival depends on the amount and size of the mixing of the two otherwise independent circulations. Patients with TGA and an intact ventricular septum present shortly after birth with cyanosis, and tend to deteriorate rapidly. When a large ventricular septal defect is present, cyanosis can be mild. Clinical presentation may be delayed by up to 2–4 weeks, and usually occurs with signs of congestive heart failure. When severe stenosis of the pulmonary artery is associated with a ventricular septal defect, symptoms are similar to those of patients with tetralogy of Fallot.

The time and mode of clinical presentation with corrected TGA depend upon the concomitant cardiac defects (ventricular septal defects, pulmonary stenosis, bradycardia, etc.).

## DOUBLE OUTLET RIGHT VENTRICLE

In double outlet right ventricle (DORV), most of the aorta and pulmonary valves arise completely or almost completely from the right ventricle. The relation between the two vessels may vary, ranging from a Fallot-like to a TGA-like situation (the Taussig–Bing anomaly). DORV is not a single malformation from a pathophysiological point of view. The term refers only to the position of the great vessels that is found in association with ventricular septal defects, tetralogy of Fallot, transposition and univentricular hearts.

The prevalence is 0.032 per 1000 live births[1]. Pulmonary stenosis is very common in all types of DORV, but left outflow obstructions, from subaortic stenosis to coarctation and interruption of the aortic arch, can also be seen.

Prenatal diagnosis of DORV can be reliably made in the fetus[13] but differentiation from other conotruncal anomalies can be very difficult, especially with tetralogy of Fallot and TGA with ventricular septal defect. The main echocardiographic features include:

(1) Alignment of the two vessels totally or predominantly from the right ventricle;

(2) Presence in most cases of bilateral coni (subaortic and subpulmonary).

The hemodynamics are dependent upon the anatomic type of DORV and the associated anomalies. Since the fetal heart works as a common chamber where the blood is mixed and pumped, the presence of DORV is not expected to be a cause of cardiac failure. Indeed, in our series of ten cases, we have never seen intrauterine heart failure. Differently from other conotruncal malformations, we have, however, frequently found extracardiac anomalies and/or chromosomal aberrations associated with fetal DORV.

## TETRALOGY OF FALLOT

The essential features of this malformation are malalignment ventricular septal defect with anterior displacement of the infundibular septum; subpulmonary narrowing and overriding aortic root; demonstrable continuity between the right outflow tract and the pulmonary trunk. In about 20% of cases, this continuity is lacking, leading to atresia of the pulmonary valve, a condition that is commonly referred to as pulmonary atresia with ventricular septal defect. Tetralogy of Fallot can be associated with other specific cardiac malformations, defining peculiar entities. These include atrioventricular septal defects, found in 4% of cases, and absence of the pulmonary valve, found in less than 2%. Hypertrophy of the right ventricle, one of the classic elements of the tetrad, is always absent in the fetus, and only develops after birth.

Echocardiographic diagnosis of tetralogy of Fallot relies upon the demonstration of a ventricular septal defect in the outlet portion of the septum and an overriding aorta (Figure 4)[2,7]. There is an inverse relationship between the size of the ascending aorta and pulmonary artery, with a disproportion that is often striking. A large aortic root is indeed an important

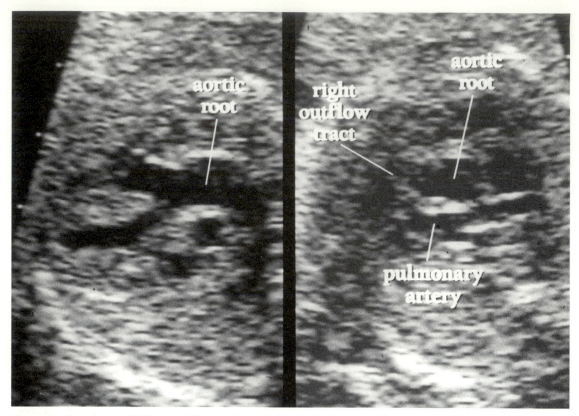

**Figure 4** Tetralogy of Fallot in a 29-week fetus. Left panel, a large aortic root is seen overriding about 50% of a defect in the ventricular septum. Right panel, short-axis view of the great vessels. The narrow outflow tract of the right ventricle and the small pulmonary artery are dwarfed by the oversized aorta. Pulsed wave Doppler ultrasound revealed increased velocities in the pulmonary artery, compatible with the diagnosis of pulmonary stenosis suggested by the bidimensional finding

diagnostic clue[14]. Doppler studies provide valuable information. The finding of increased peak velocities in the pulmonary artery corroborates the diagnosis of tetralogy of Fallot by suggesting obstruction to blood flow in the right outflow tract. Conversely, demonstration with color and/or pulsed Doppler that in the pulmonary artery there is either no forward flow or reverse flow allows a diagnosis of pulmonary atresia.

Diagnostic problems arise at the extremes of the spectrum of tetralogy of Fallot. In cases with minor forms of right outflow obstruction and aortic overriding, differentiation from a simple ventricular septal defect can be difficult. In those cases in which the pulmonary artery is not imaged, a differential diagnosis between pulmonary atresia with ventricular septal defect and

truncus arteriosus communis is similarly difficult.

The sonographer should also be alerted to a frequent artefact that resembles overriding of the aorta. Incorrect orientation of the transducer may demonstrate apparent septo-aortic discontinuity in a normal fetus. The mechanism of the artefact is probably related to the angle of incidence of the sound beam. Albeit such an artefact caused the only false-positive diagnosis in our series[4], our further experience suggests that careful visualization of the left outflow tract with different insonation angles, as well as the use of color Doppler and the research of the other elements of the tetralogy, should virtually eliminate this problem.

Atrioventricular connections need to be carefully assessed to rule out the possible association with atrioventricular septal defects. Such a combination is associated with an increased risk of concomitant autosomal trisomies, Down's syndrome in particular[15,16], and results *per se* in a worse prognosis. Abnormal enlargement of the right ventricle, main pulmonary trunk and artery suggests absence of the pulmonary valve[2].

Evaluation of other variables, such as multiple ventricular septal defects and coronary anomalies, would be valuable for a better prediction of surgical timing and operative prognosis. Unfortunately, these findings cannot be recognized for certain by prenatal echocardiography at present.

Cardiac failure is never seen in fetal life as well as postnatally. Even in cases of tight pulmonary stenosis or atresia, the wide ventricular septal defect provides adequate combined ventricular output, while the pulmonary vascular bed is supplied in a retrograde manner by the ductus. The only exception to this rule is represented by cases with an absent pulmonary valve that may result in massive regurgitation to the right ventricle and atrium.

When severe pulmonic stenosis is present, cyanosis tends to develop immediately after birth. When a lesser degree of obstruction to pulmonary blood flow is present, the onset of cyanosis may not appear until later in the first year of life. When there is pulmonary atresia, rapid and severe deterioration follows ductal constriction.

## TRUNCUS ARTERIOSUS COMMUNIS

Truncus arteriosus is characterized by a single arterial vessel that originates from the heart, overrides the ventricular septum and supplies the systemic, pulmonary and coronary circulations.

The single arterial trunk is larger than the normal aortic root and is predominantly connected with the right ventricle in roughly 42% of cases, with the left ventricle in 16%, and is equally shared in 42%[17]. The truncal valve may have one, two or three cusps and is rarely normal. It can be stenotic or, more frequently, insufficient. A malalignment ventricular septal defect, usually wide, is an essential part of the malformation.

Truncus arteriosus can be classified in different, similar ways, according to Collett and Edwards[18] and Van Praagh and Van Praagh[19]. The following situations can be recognized:

(1) The pulmonary arteries arise from the truncus within a short distance from the valve, as a main pulmonary trunk which then bifurcates (type A or I) or without the main pulmonary trunk (type A2 or II and III); and

(2) Less frequently, only one pulmonary artery (usually the right) originates from the truncus while the other is supplied by a systemic collateral vessel from the descending aorta (type A3).

Truncus is associated with interrupted aortic arch (type A4) in 11% of cases. Similar to tetralogy of Fallot, and unlike the other conotruncal malformations, truncus is frequently associated with extracardiac malformations, in a proportion ranging between 20 and 40%.

Truncus arteriosus can be reliably detected with fetal echocardiography (Figures 5 and 6). The main diagnostic criteria are a single semilunar valve overriding the ventricular septal defect and a direct continuity existing between one or two pulmonary arteries and the single arterial trunk.

The semilunar valve is often thickened and moves abnormally. Doppler ultrasound is of value to assess incompetence of the truncal valve.

A peculiar problem found in prenatal echocardiography is the demonstration of the absence of pulmonary outflow tract and the concomitant failure to image the pulmonary arteries. In this situation, a differentiation between truncus and pulmonary atresia with ventricular septal defect may be impossible.

Similar to the other conotruncal anomalies, truncus arteriosus is not associated with alteration of fetal hemodynamics. The only remarkable exception is the case with an incompetent truncal valve, that may result in massive regurgitation of blood to the ventricles and

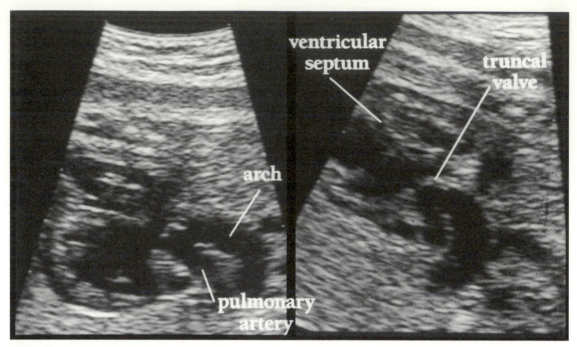

**Figure 5** Truncus arteriosus type A. Left panel, a single large vessel is seen arising from the base of the heart. A common pulmonary artery originates posteriorly from the arterial trunk. Right panel, a close-up of the truncus arteriosus demonstrates a large and thickened truncal valve. The aorto-pulmonary septum is seen dividing distally the truncus into its aortic and pulmonary portions.

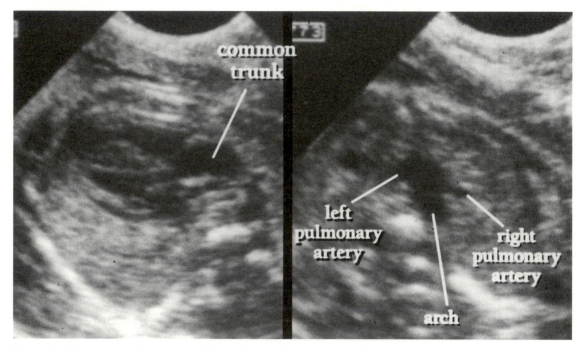

**Figure 6** Truncus arteriosus, type A2 in a 29-week fetus. Left panel, a single large vessel is seen arising from the base of the heart, overriding a ventricular septal defect. Right panel, the single vessel is identified as a truncus arteriosus by demonstrating that it gives origin to both pulmonary arteries and to the aortic arch

cause congestive heart failure. This, however, has never happened in our series of five consecutive cases, neither are we aware of any such case reported in the literature. Truncus arteriosus is frequently a neonatal emergency. These patients usually have unobstructed pulmonary blood flow and show signs of progressive congestive heart failure with the postnatal fall in pulmonary resistance. Many patients will present with cardiac failure in the first 1 or 2 weeks of life.

## ANTENATAL DIAGNOSIS OF CONOTRUNCAL ANOMALIES: PERSONAL EXPERIENCE

From 1981 to 1994, we observed a total of 174 fetal cardiac malformations, mainly from investigation of a high-risk obstetric population. Of these, 44 (26%) were conotruncal abnormalities (Table 1). Extracardiac malformations and/or chromosomal aberrations were present in four of these cases (9%). Congestive heart failure never occurred *in utero*.

In most cases, the antenatal echocardiographic diagnosis was found to be correct, albeit prior to the introduction of Duplex ultrasound the antenatal identification of pulmonary atresia was uncertain. There was only one error, that occurred at the very beginning of our experience (one false-positive diagnosis of tetralogy of Fallot), and five imprecisions that did not affect perinatal management: in one case of complete TGA with associated ventricular septal defect and pulmonary stenosis, the antenatal diagnosis was double outlet right ventricle; in one fetus with multiple anomalies and oligohydramnios, complete TGA was diagnosed echocardiographically and a rare form of double outlet left ventricle was recognized after birth; in one case of tetralogy of Fallot with mild right

**Table 1** Prenatal diagnosis of fetal cardiac malformations at Bologna University School of Medicine between 1981 and 1994

| | |
|---|---|
| Simple defects | 48 |
| Univentricular hearts | 32 |
| Hypoplasia of left ventricle | 26 |
| Conotruncal anomalies | 44 |
|   tetralogy of Fallot/pulmonary atresia with VSD | 20 |
|   double outlet right ventricle | 10 |
|   complete TGA | 6 |
|   corrected TGA | 2 |
|   truncus | 5 |
|   double outlet left ventricle | 1 |
| Others, complex | 24 |
| Total | 174 |

TGA, transposition of great arteries; VSD, ventricular septal defect

outflow obstruction, only a ventricular septal defect was identified *in utero*. Eventually, in two cases, the differentiation between truncus arteriosus and pulmonary atresia with ventricular septal defects could only be made after birth.

## CONCLUSIONS

Conotruncal anomalies are amenable to accurate antenatal echocardiographic diagnosis from early stages of fetal development. Meticulous scanning is required, however, and the recognition of the specific type of anomaly is difficult at times. In the overall majority of cases, these defects do not cause hemodynamic compromise of the fetal circulation and allow normal intrauterine development. Prenatal recognition may be beneficial, as the onset of symptoms is often dramatic after birth. Prompt treatment of these otherwise severe conditions allows long-term survival, with normal growth and development in most cases.

# References

1. Fyler, D. C. (1980). Report of the New England Regional Cardiac Program. *Pediatrics*, **65** (Suppl.), 375–461

2. Kleinman, C. S., Donnerstein, R. L., DeVore, G. R., Jaffe, C. C., Lynch, D. C., Berkowitz, R. L., Talner, L. S. and Hobbins, J. C. (1982). Fetal echocardiography for evaluation of *in utero* congestive heart failure. *N. Engl. J. Med.*, **306**, 568–75

3. Allan, L. D., Crawford, D. C., Andersen, R. H. and Tynan, M. J. (1984). Echocardiographic and anatomical correlates in fetal congenital heart disease. *Br. Heart J.*, **52**, 542–8

4. Pilu, G. and Baccarani, G. (1986). Prenatal diagnosis of cardiac structural abnormalities. *Fetal Ther.*, **1**, 86–7

5. Copel, J. A., Pilu, G., Greene, J., Hobbins, J. C. and Kleinman, C. S. (1987). Fetal echocardiographic screening for congenital heart disease: the importance of the four-chamber view. *Am. J. Obstet. Gynecol.*, **157**, 648–52

6. Davis, G. K., Farquhar, C. M., Allan, L. D., Crawford, D. C. and Chapman, M. G. (1990). Structural cardiac abnormalities in the fetus: reliability of prenatal diagnosis and outcome. *Br. J. Obstet. Gynaecol.*, **97**, 27–31

7. Sanders, S. P., Bierman, F. Z. and Williams, R. G. (1982). Conotruncal malformations: diagnosis in infancy using subxiphoid 2-dimensional echocardiography. *Am. J. Cardiol.*, **50**, 1361–7

8. Allan, L. D., Tynan, M. J., Wilkinson, J. L. and Anderson, R. H. (1980). Echocardiographic and anatomical correlates in the fetus. *Br. Heart J.*, **40**, 441–51

9. Gembruch, U., Knopfle, G., Bald, R. and Hansmann, M. (1993). Early diagnosis of congenital heart disease by transvaginal echocardiography. *Ultrasound Obstet. Gynecol.*, **3**, 310–17

10. DeVore, G. R. (1994). Color Doppler examination of the outflow tracts of the fetal heart: a technique for identification of cardiovascular malformations. *Ultrasound Obstet. Gynecol.*, **4**, 463–71

11. Becker, A. E. and Anderson, R H. (1981). *Pathology of Congenital Heart Disease*. (London: Butterworths)

12. Schmidt, K. G., Ulmer, H. E., Silverman, N. H., Kleinman, C. S. and Copel, J. A. (1991). Perinatal outcome of fetal complete atrioventricular block: a multicenter experience. *J. Am. Coll. Cardiol.*, **17**, 1360–6

13. Stewart, P. A., Wladimiroff, J. W. and Becker, A. E. (1985). Early prenatal detection of double outlet right ventricle by echocardiography. *Br. Heart J.*, **54**, 340–2

14. DeVore, G. R., Siassi, B. and Platt, L. D. (1988). Fetal echocardiography VIII. Aortic root dilatation – a marker for tetralogy of Fallot. *Am. J. Obstet. Gynecol.*, **159**, 129–36

15. Copel, J. A., Pilu, G. and Kleinman, C. S. (1986). Congenital heart disease and extra-cardiac malformations. Associations and indications for fetal echocardiography. *Am. J. Obstet. Gynecol.*, **154**, 1121–30

16. Rizzo, N., Pittalis, M. C., Pilu, G., Orsini, L. F., Perolo, A. and Bovicelli, L. (1990). Prenatal karyotyping in malformed fetuses. *Prenat. Diagn.*, **10**, 17–21

17. Hernanz-Schulman, M. and Fellows, K. E. (1985). Persistent truncus arteriosus: pathologic, diagnostic and therapeutical considerations. *Semin. Roentgenol.*, **20**, 121–9

18. Collett, R. W. and Edwards, J. E. (1949). Persistent truncus arteriosus. A classification according to anatomic types. *Surg. Clin. North. Am.*, **29**, 1245–70

19. Van Praagh, R. and Van Praagh, S. (1965). The anatomy of common aorticopulmonary trunk (truncus arteriosus communis) and its embryologic implications. A study of 57 necropsy cases. *Am. J. Cardiol.*, **16**, 406–21

# Routine screening for congenital heart disease: a prospective study in the Netherlands

7

*E. Buskens, D. E. Grobbee, J. W. Wladimiroff and J. Hess*

## INTRODUCTION

Congenital heart disease constitutes an important proportion of all major congenital malformations, which are present in 2–3% of neonates[1,2]. The estimated birth prevalence of cardiac malformations is 8 per 1000[3]. Approximately half of the cases of congenital heart disease have only minor consequences or can easily be corrected surgically. Yet, 35% of the infant deaths due to congenital malformations are related to cardiovascular anomalies[4,5]. Hence, congenital heart disease is still an important issue in infant health. In addition, cardiovascular anomalies are strongly associated with other anomalies or chromosomal aberrations[6–8].

At present, the etiology of congenital heart disease is to a large extent unknown. Approximately 90% of the cases are of multifactorial origin, e.g. result from an interaction between genetic constitution and environmental influences without further etiological specification[9]. Accordingly, the majority of affected infants are born to mothers without previously known risk factors for bearing children with congenital heart disease. This implies that most of the severe cases will become apparent at or soon after birth unless detected prenatally. A systematic prenatal screening procedure for congenital malformations of the heart made available to all pregnant women may quicken the diagnosis of such an affliction to a point in time which allows adjustment of obstetric management[10,11]. Over the last decades, diagnostic ultrasound examination of the human fetus has evolved from a research tool into a valuable clinical diagnostic test. Congenital heart disease

has proven to be accessible for prenatal detection in many cases[12–21]. Generally, it is assumed that this in turn could have beneficial effects for the neonate and the parent(s). The timing, location and the mode of delivery can be determined to grant the neonate optimal chances for survival[22–24]. The strong association with chromosomal defects and non-cardiac malformations implies that karyotyping and extended structural ultrasound examination of the fetus should be performed after detection of an anomaly[6,7,25,26]. Subsequently, genetic counselling can be offered to the parents to inform them of the risk they carry for having affected offspring in the future. In cases of fetal tachycardia, possibly associated with fetal hydrops, transplacental drug treatment may be offered to try and improve fetal condition[27–29]. The recent development of fetal medicine has created a new era of possibilities. Furthermore, detecting a non-viable fetus early in pregnancy offers the option of termination of pregnancy. Eventually, reassuring the future parents after having excluded (severe) fetal anomalies may be perceived as the greatest benefit of screening.

Many reports have appeared on the efficacy of ultrasound screening for congenital heart disease in obstetrics[13,15,16,20,21,30–34]. The majority, however, originate from teaching hospitals or tertiary referral institutions with above average expertise and interest in the subject. Also, interpretation of the results obtained is sometimes hampered because of variability in study design. Additionally, and perhaps more importantly, the patients involved may be a selection

71

of high-risk cases. Accordingly, as we have recently shown that the findings of experts may not be representative for a routine screening program[35], a prospective study on routine fetal ultrasound screening in the Netherlands will be presented.

## A PROSPECTIVE STUDY IN THE NETHERLANDS

Assessment of the four-chamber view has been incorporated into 'routine' fetal ultrasound in many countries including the Netherlands[36]. In spite of its popularity, a formal evaluation of the routine ultrasound examination of the fetal heart by means of the fetal four-chamber view performed once in a low-risk population at a gestational age of about 20 weeks has, to our knowledge, not been performed.

## SUBJECTS AND METHODS

### Source population

Pregnant women referred for routine fetal ultrasound were considered eligible if scheduled for routine fetal ultrasound between 16 and 24 weeks of pregnancy. Determination of gestational age or growth discrepancy, reassurance because of a preceding miscarriage, lack of fetal movements, inability to detect fetal heart beats and some miscellaneous reasons were also considered a routine examination. All women with known risk factors for congenital heart disease in their offspring, e.g. a previous child, their partner or themselves affected with congenital heart disease, maternal juvenile diabetes, maternal lupus erythematosus, maternal phenyl ketonuria, maternal rubella and maternal drug or teratogen exposure, for example use of anticonvulsants, retinoic acid or morphomimetics, were excluded as these characteristics currently constitute an acknowledged indication for additional fetal echocardiography. The women were invited to participate in the study by the sonographers, e.g. ultrasound technicians, midwives, or physicians. Together, 15 referring ultrasound units in the Rotterdam metropolitan area participated. All participating women reside in the

south-western part of the Netherlands. From March 1991 until January 1993, 6922 fetuses were scanned and included in the study. Mean maternal age was 28.9 years (SD 4.6; range 14–47).

### Personnel and appliances

In each of the participating ultrasound centers, the majority of examinations was performed by specific experienced personnel. Technicians performed the majority of scans, 3747 (54%) in total. Midwives performed 776 (11%), trainees in obstetrics and gynecology 1391 (20%) and consultants 1008 (15%). The majority of sonographers involved in the study had ample background in fetal ultrasound examination including an intensive 2-day ultrasound training course on the evaluation of the fetal four-chamber view. Various brands and types of ultrasound equipment, all state-of-the-art two-dimensional appliances, were used in the participating ultrasound units depending on local preference. The study was intended to investigate a setting that resembled routine practice as closely as possible with regard to experience and expertise of the sonographers as well as quality of equipment.

### Data handling

All ultrasound examinations of the fetal four-chamber view were evaluated and coded as normal, abnormal or impossible to assess, according to standard criteria. The fetal heart should be located in the middle of the thorax, occupy approximately one-third of the thorax, display atria of equal size, ventricles of equal size, an intact ventricular septum, a foramen ovale flap demonstrated in the left atrium and have off-set atrioventricular valves, that is, a more apical insertion of the tricuspid valve and possible visualization of a 'moderator band' in the right ventricle[13,16] (Figure 1). In addition, data on gestational age as determined by biometry, a code for the category of referring obstetrician (midwife, general practitioner, or gynecologist) and the indication for an ultrasound scan (routine, determination of gestational age or

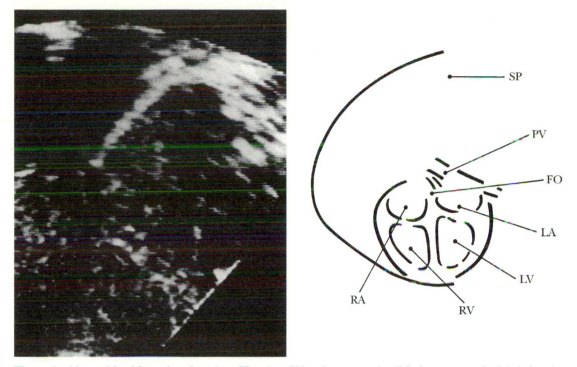

**Figure 1**  Normal fetal four-chamber view: SP, spine; PV, pulmonary veins; FO, foramen ovale; LA, left atrium; LV, left ventricle; RV, right ventricle; RA, right atrium

other) were recorded. Finally, non-cardiac malformation(s) suspected (according to guidelines issued by the Netherlands Society for Obstetrics and Gynecology[36]) and whether or not the pregnant woman was subsequently referred for extended fetal ultrasound examination, were registered. Follow-up data on all women and their children were collected until 6 months postnatally. In collaboration with local Child Health Clinics, which offer a physical examination of the infants and an interview of the parents at monthly intervals from birth onwards, the required data (date of birth, sex and presence of congenital anomalies) were obtained for most women. In cases where an anomaly was suspected and the infant was referred, hospital records, findings on additional ultrasound examination and autopsy records were retrieved and coded.

## Data analysis

By comparing the prenatal diagnosis (presence or absence of anomalies) to the postnatal diagnosis, the latter being taken as a gold standard, all ultrasound examinations were categorized as true positive where a suspected anomaly was confirmed, false positive where a suspected anomaly could not be confirmed, false negative where an anomaly was missed by ultrasound examination, or true negative where no anomalies were present. As no consequences are attached to a four-chamber view examination that appeared to be indeterminable, the cases involved were considered to have a normal screening test. The data were subdivided according to the presence of congenital heart disease and non-cardiac congenital anomalies. In addition, all anomalies were categorized as major (definitely considered detectable prenatally, e.g. disrupting four-chamber anatomy), minor (possibility of prenatal detection is debatable due to size or type of anomaly), or undetectable (excluded from analysis, e.g. patent arterial duct or open foramen ovale). As there is general consensus that the latter anomalies can be considered part of normal fetal development or cannot be recognized on prenatal ultrasound examination these cases were subsequently omitted from analysis[37]. The sensitivity, the specificity, the positive predictive value and the negative predictive value were calculated with corresponding exact 95% binomial confidence intervals[40]. In addition, the prevalence of congenital malformations (the proportion of infants affected) was calculated.

## RESULTS

### Subjects and ultrasound examinations

Of the total of 6922 fetuses screened, 6571 (95%) underwent a routine ultrasound examination between 16 and 24 weeks' gestational age. Figure 2 shows the distribution of the duration of pregnancy at which the ultrasound examinations were performed. In 501 (7.2%) fetuses, an adequate four-chamber view could not be obtained. Figure 2 also demonstrates how visualization of the four-chamber view related to gestational age. Follow-up until 6 months postpartum has been completed for 5660 fetuses (81.8%). Of these, 119 appeared to have been included despite known risk factors for congenital heart disease and 222 were screened outside the 16–24 weeks' gestational age range. Consequently, the analysis presented pertains to 5319 routine fetal ultrasound examinations in the gestational age range of 16–24 weeks (mean

19 weeks and 5 days), with complete information available on the outcome of pregnancy until 6 months postpartum.

### Outcome of ultrasound

Of all women screened prenatally, seven subjects (0.10%) were subsequently referred for extended fetal echocardiography on account of an abnormal appearance of the fetal four-chamber view. Another 14 (0.20%) subjects were referred because of other suspected congenital anomalies. Two cases of intrauterine referral for suspected congenital heart disease could be confirmed on subsequent evaluation. Non-cardiac anomalies were detected more accurately; out of the 14 cases referred, 12 proved to be affected.

### Outcome of pregnancy

Eventually, congenital anomalies were recognized in 118 (2.2%; 95% confidence interval 1.8–2.7) cases. There were 62 (1.2%; 0.9–1.5) cases with congenital heart disease (six of which also had other congenital anomalies). Non-cardiac anomalies were detected in 62 (1.2%; 0.9–1.5) cases. Furthermore, five cases of congenital heart disease occurred in combination with chromosomal anomalies. When evaluated

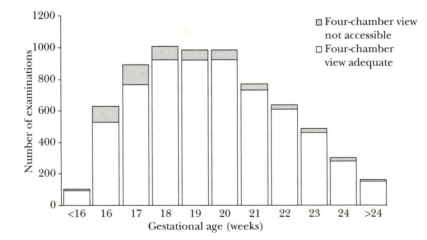

**Figure 2** Distribution of gestational age at the time of ultrasound examination with proportional display of adequate four-chamber view evaluations

according to categories (major, minor, or unrecognizable) of anomalies, 80 (1.5%; 1.2–1.9) major and minor cases remained for secondary analysis. These included 44 cases of congenital heart disease (four in combination with other malformations), and 40 cases of non-cardiac anomalies. The nature of the congenital anomalies encountered in these 80 cases is listed and categorized according to detectability and organ system or structure in Table 1. As any one fetus or infant may have more than one anomaly, over 80 anomalies are listed.

## Performance of ultrasound

In the categories of cardiac anomalies, non-cardiac anomalies and all anomalies combined, a distinction has been made between the number of major and minor anomalies together and the subsample of major anomalies likely to have generated an abnormal image at 20 weeks' gestational age. This is reflected in separate tables and analyses according to case severity. Table 2 shows the findings of routine prenatal screening for congenital anomalies of the heart, non-cardiac anomalies and all anomalies combined, respectively. The sensitivity for cases of congenital heart disease was low (5%; 0.6–15) even if only major anomalies were considered (17%; 2.1–49). Sensitivity was somewhat higher for

non-cardiac anomalies (30%; 17–47) and higher still in case of major anomalies (40%; 23–59). The sensitivity for all anomalies combined was intermediate (overall: 16%; 9–26, major: 33%; 19–50). As expected, the specificity was high (> 99%) for both categories of anomalies. Also, the negative predictive value was high (99%). The positive predictive value varied con-

**Table 1** Congenital anomalies detected in 80 cases during follow-up with numbers detected prenatally in parentheses

|  | Total | Major |
|---|---|---|
| Ventricular septal defect | 30 | 4 |
| Coarctation of the aorta | 5 | |
| Atrioventricular septal defect | 4 | 4 |
| Atrial septal defect | 5 | |
| Pulmonary atresia | 4 | |
| Pulmonary stenosis | 2 | |
| Transposition of the great arteries | 2 | |
| Hypoplastic left heart | 1 | 1 |
| Hypoplastic right heart | 1 | 1 |
| Double outlet right ventricle | 1 | |
| Complex cardiac anomalies | 2 | 2 (2) |
| Urogenital | 11 | 4 (3) |
| Gastrointestinal | 6 | 5 (3) |
| Extremities | 8 | 8 |
| Facial | 8 | 4 |
| Central nervous system | 3 | 2 |
| Miscellaneous | 6 | 6 (5) |

**Table 2** Outcome of ultrasound screening for congenital anomalies and findings on follow-up

|  | Anomalies* | Normal | Major anomalies | Normal | Total |
|---|---|---|---|---|---|
| Congenital heart disease | | | | | |
| abnormal four-chamber view | 2 | 5 | 2 | 5 | 7 |
| normal four-chamber view | 42 | 5270 | 10 | 5302 | 5312 |
| total | 44 (18)[†] (3)[‡] | 5275 | 12 | 5307 | 5319 |
| Non-cardiac malformations | | | | | |
| non-cardiac screen positive | 12 | 2 | 12 | 2 | 14 |
| non-cardiac screen negative | 28 | 5277 | 18 | 5287 | 5305 |
| total | 40 (22)[†] | 5279 | 30 | 5289 | 5319 |
| All anomalies combined | | | | | |
| screen positive | 13 (1)[§] | 7 | 13 | 7 | 20 |
| screen negative | 67 (3)[§] (2)[¶] | 5232 | 26 | 5273 | 5299 |
| total | 80 (38)[†] | 5239 | 39 | 5280 | 5319 |

*Major and minor anomalies; [†]cases not included; non-detectable anomalies; [‡]non-detectable cardiovascular anomalies but detectable non-cardiac anomalies; [§]number of cases with both cardiac and non-cardiac anomalies; [¶]major anomalies

siderably over the categories of anomalies and could not be established accurately, as illustrated by the wide confidence intervals. All test characteristics and prevalence figures are summarized in Table 3.

## Validation

As the possibility of selective participation of women with fetuses that have no anomalies or, alternatively, a relatively high number of anomalies, was a major concern, a random sample of 1500 ultrasound examinations (100 from each of the participating ultrasound units) was evaluated with regard to data on gestational age, referring obstetrician, indication of ultrasound, suspected presence of congenital malformations and referral for further evaluation. Because this random sample could not be selected on gestational age a wider gestational age, range is represented. Also, it appeared that slightly more examinations in the sample were requested by consultants. However, the (small) proportion of women referred on account of suspected fetal anomalies was equal to that in the study population. In addition, the database of the Division of Prenatal Diagnosis of the Department of Obstetrics and Gynecology of Dijkzigt University Hospital, serving the Rotterdam metropolitan area as a tertiary referral center, could be checked for cases not included in the study that would otherwise have qualified as participants. During the period of intake, only one case of a suspected anomaly of the fetal four-chamber had been referred that was not known from the regular follow-up.

## INTERPRETATION OF THE DATA

The objective of the study described was to evaluate the efficacy of the fetal four-chamber view in routine screening of normal pregnancies to detect congenital heart disease. The findings indicate that the fetal four-chamber view, as evaluated during routine fetal ultrasound in the second trimester of pregnancy, does not provide an accurate screening test. Even major anomalies, likely to create an abnormal fetal four-chamber view, were not detected to a satisfactory degree prenatally.

Several factors may explain these results. The size of the fetal structures is related to gestational age. Hence, visualization early in the second trimester, when the fetus is small, will be limited by the resolution of the ultrasound equipment. However, as is apparent from Figure 2, the majority of scans was performed beyond 17 weeks' gestational age, a time generally deemed appropriate for structural ultrasound examination. In addition, the proportion of fetal hearts that could not be assessed remained stable after 17 weeks of gestation; the scans appear to have been performed at an appropriate moment. Furthermore, all participating ultrasound units had state-of-the-art equipment at their disposal. Conversely, other factors may be responsible for the results. The scans were performed by specialized technicians, midwives, or consultants trained in ultrasound examination in 80% of the cases and by sonographers (trainees) with varying degrees of experience in the remainder of the group. This mix, however, adequately reflects the current ultrasound practice of routine screening. In ad-

**Table 3** Test characteristics of routine fetal ultrasound

|  | Cardiac anomalies | | Other congenital anomalies | | Overall | |
| --- | --- | --- | --- | --- | --- | --- |
| Sensitivity | | | | | | |
| major and minor | 5 | (0.6–15) | 30 | (17–47) | 16 | (9–26) |
| major | 17 | (2–49) | 40 | (23–59) | 33 | (19–50) |
| Specificity | 99.9 | (99.8–100) | 99.9 | (99.9–100) | 99.9 | (99.7–100) |
| Positive predictive value | 29 | (3.7–71) | 86 | (57–98) | 65 | (41–85) |
| Negative predictive value | 99.2 | (98.9–99.4) | 99.5 | (99.2–99.7) | 98.7 | (98.4–99.0) |
| Prevalence | | | | | | |
| major and minor | 0.8 | (0.6–1.1) | 0.8 | (0.5–1.0) | 1.5 | (1.2–1.9) |
| all cases | 1.2 | (0.9–1.5) | 1.2 | (0.9–1.5) | 2.2 | (1.8–2.7) |

All figures are % with 95% confidence intervals in parentheses

dition, all participating ultrasound units were visited regularly to verify the progress of the study and assess the demand for additional training of junior sonographers. By evaluating the number of inadequate four-chamber view visualizations during the study, the effect of increasing experience of the sonographers can be judged. However, the proportion of adequate ultrasound evaluations of the fetal heart did not materially fluctuate nor was there any indication of a particular trend during the period of participation. Interestingly, the proportion of fetal four-chamber views judged as indeterminable did not differ among the categories of sonographers. Furthermore, all sonographers had taken similar additional training in the fetal four-chamber view examination prior to the start of participation in the study. Accordingly, it appears unlikely that variation in experience and skills has had a major impact on the efficacy of the screening procedure. For non-cardiac congenital anomalies also, a rather poor performance was observed with a 30% sensitivity, resulting in a sensitivity of 16% for all anomalies together. A discussion analogous to that on the fetal four-chamber view applies to other congenital anomalies as well. Again, the results cannot be readily explained by any of the variables discussed so far.

The nature of the anomalies encountered in routine screening may explain part of the low sensitivity of prenatal detection observed in this study. Some malformations, for instance a small ventricular septal defect or an atrial septal defect, may not be visible with the current ultrasound equipment or may not be visible by means of the four-chamber view alone. The proportional distribution of congenital anomalies encountered at birth may clarify this argument. Thirty per cent of the cases have ventricular septal defects, 10% have a patent ductus arteriosus, 10% have atrial septal defects, 10% have pulmonary stenosis and a further 25% are cases of tetralogy of Fallot, coarctation of the aorta, aortic stenosis and transposition of the great arteries[39]. It can be argued that approximately half may not be detectable (or only with great difficulty) by means of a fetal four-chamber view. Furthermore, a congenital anomaly may not

remain in a steady state. A duodenal obstruction, or a urinary tract obstruction for instance, may only become visible in the late second trimester. The anatomical substrate may be present already, but may not yet have functional (recognizable) consequences at 20 weeks' gestation. This may even apply in some severe cardiac anomalies like hypoplastic left heart[40]. Specific conditions of the ultrasound examination may add a further explanation for the failure to recognize even gross cardiac pathology. Severe maternal obesity or unfavorable fetal position may considerably hamper the possibilities to assess the fetal structures. However, the stable and limited proportion of cases with an indeterminable four-chamber view does not support a major effect of scanning conditions. Apparently, the sensitivity is partly determined by the (im)possibilities of detection by means of prenatal ultrasound and partly by the natural history of the specific anomalies. Nevertheless, even if anomalies of which possibilities for prenatal detection are debatable were left out of the analysis, low sensitivities were found. Excluding 'minor' anomalies from evaluation could suggest that one considers these cases irrelevant from an obstetric and pediatric point of view. Yet, minor variants of congenital malformations may have an identical cause as major defects and may similarly be associated with other anomalies. In view of this it would seem irrational to consider such cases irrelevant.

## COMPARISON WITH OTHER STUDIES

As mentioned above, fetal four-chamber view screening has been advocated as a useful tool with which to detect congenital heart disease prenatally[13,16]. Apparently, the data from the Dutch prospective study are not consistent with this view. The reports published, however, mostly originate from experts in the field of fetal ultrasound who tend to work in (tertiary) referral centers. For instance, Vergani and co-workers[34] reported a sensitivity of 81%. This was achieved in a referral hospital with at least one scan performed at varying gestational age, in a mixed high- and low-risk population. Furthermore, postnatal follow-up was not ascertained beyond 1 week postnatally, which may have caused an underestimation of the prevalence and, subsequently, an overestimation of the sensitivity. The results are likely not to apply to the routine ultrasound clinic, where sonographers may be less skilled, face crowded office hours and a non-selected population with a low prevalence of anomalies. In addition, the Dutch prospective cohort study has complete follow-up on the fetuses, whereas previous reports are limited to cases referred and detected. This may have caused a serious bias. Stillborn fetuses or infants affected may not reach (a tertiary) hospital or may not be examined routinely. When such false-negative cases are not considered, this will result in overestimated sensitivities. Recent reports on ultrasound in second-trimester pregnancy, originating from ultrasound units employing typical personnel and scanning time, show an efficacy of routine fetal ultrasound examination for detection of congenital anomalies, and cardiac anomalies in particular, that is compatible with our findings[41–46].

As discussed, the level of expertise and skills of the sonographers in the Dutch study represents the level of quality in ultrasound examination usually observed in routine screening practice. Suggestions for additional training of the sonographers as well as additional scanning projections have been submitted[47,48]. However, great endeavor and substantial resources may be required to establish a level of ultrasound skills sufficient to have a major impact on detection rates. Even if achieved, a sizable proportion of cases may remain technically undetectable within the period of gestational age considered optimal for screening. Despite obvious advantages of prenatal detection of individual cases, an overall net benefit of routine ultrasound screening for cardiac anomalies could not be established. False-negative diagnoses and false-positive diagnoses will always occur and have to be taken into account. In addition, it may well be that, in a major proportion of the cases potentially detectable, prognosis will not improve significantly by early detection[49,50].

In conclusion, the findings in the prospective Dutch study described indicate that routine fetal echocardiography at 20 weeks' gestational age by means of the fetal four-chamber view at present does not suffice as a prenatal screening test for congenital heart disease. A recent paper by our group, on the hypothetical yield a high-quality routine screening program might have, indicates that only a small impact on infant morbidity and mortality may be obtained[51]. According to the best available estimates of the test characteristics of prenatal screening for congenital heart disease by means of the fetal four-chamber view, the yield, expressed as the prevention of the birth of a critically ill neonate, appears to be numerically modest.

## ACKNOWLEDGEMENTS

We are very much indebted to all pregnant women, sonographers, obstetricians, child health clinics, general practitioners, pediatricians and pediatric cardiologists for their willingness to co-operate and provide us with the necessary data. In addition, we thank Andrina Cleveringa, Sharmila Bhikha and Agnes van der Voorn for their enthusiastic and skilful contribution to the data collection and management and Marcel Eijgermans for his continuous support regarding data-base handling. The study was supported by a research grant (NHS 98.053) from the Netherlands Heart Foundation.

# References

1. Cornel, M. C., de Walle, H. E. K., Haveman, T. M., Spreen, J. A., Breed, A. C. and ten Kate, L. P. (1991). Birth prevalence of congenital anomalies in the Northern Netherlands. (Prevalentie van meer dan 30 aangeboren afwijkingen

in Noord-Nederland.) *Ned. Tijdschr. Geneesk.*, **135**, 2032–6

2. Holmes, L. B. (1979). Congenital malformations. In Vaughan, V. C., McKay, R. J. Behrman, R. E. and Nelson, W. E. (eds.) *Nelson. Textbook of Pediatrics.* 11th edn. p. 370. (Philadelphia: W. B. Saunders Company)

3. Campbell, M. (1973). Incidence of cardiac malformations at birth and later, and neonatal mortality. *Br. Heart J.*, **35**, 189–200

4. Central Bureau of Statistics. Ministry of Welfare, Health and Cultural Affairs (1980). *Mortality tables: Central Bureau of Statistics. Compendium of Health Statistics of the Netherlands 1986.* 's-Gravenhage: Staatsdrukkerij

5. Keith, J. D. (1978). Prevalence, incidence, and epidemiology. In Keith, J. D., Rowe, R. D. and Vlad, P. (eds.) *Heart Disease in Infancy and Childhood*, pp. 3–13. (New York: MacMillan Publishing Co.)

6. Copel, J. A., Cullen, M., Green, J. J., Mahoney, M. J., Hobbins, J. C. and Kleinman, C. S. (1988). The frequency of aneuploidy in prenatally diagnosed congenital heart disease: an indication for fetal karyotyping. *Am. J. Obstet. Gynecol.*, **158**, 409–13

7. Nora, J. J. and Hart-Nora, A. (1984). The genetic contribution to congenital heart diseases. In Nora, J. J. and Takao, A. (eds.) *Congenital Heart Disease: Causes and Processes*, pp. 3–13. (Mount Kisko, New York: Futura Publishing Co.)

8. Wladimiroff, J. W., Stewart, P. A., Sachs, E. S. and Niermeijer, M. F. (1985). Prenatal diagnosis and management of congenital heart defect: significance of associated fetal anomalies and prenatal chromosome studies. *Am. J. Med. Genet.*, **21**, 285–90

9. Nora, J. J. and Hart-Nora, A. (1984). The environmental contribution to congenital heart diseases. In Nora, J. J. and Takao, A. (eds.) *Congenital Heart Disease: Causes and Processes* pp. 15–27. (Mount Kisko, New York: Futura Publishing Co.)

10. Chang, A. C., Huhta, J. C., Yoon, G. Y. *et al.* (1991). Diagnosis, transport, and outcome in fetuses with left ventricular outflow tract obstruction. *J. Thorac. Cardiovasc. Surg.*, **102**, 841–8

11. Crawford, D. C., Chita, S. K. and Allan, L. D. (1988). Prenatal detection of congenital heart disease: factors affecting obstetric management and survival. *Am. J. Obstet. Gynecol.*, **159**, 352–6

12. Allan, L. D., Crawford, D. C., Anderson, R. H. and Tynan, M. J. (1984). Echocardiographic and anatomical correlations in fetal congenital heart disease. *Br. Heart J.*, **52**, 542–8

13. Allan, L. D., Crawford, D. C., Chita, S. K. and Tynan, M. J. (1980). Prenatal screening for congenital heart disease. *Br. Med. J.*, (*Clin. Res. Ed.*), **292**, 1717–19

14. Benacerraf, B. R. and Sanders, S. P. (1990). Fetal echocardiography. *Radiol. Clin. North Am.*, **28**, 131–47

15. Bromley, B., Estroff, J. A., Sanders, S. P., Parad, R., Roberts, D., Frigoletto, F. D. Jr and Benacerraf, B. R. (1992). Fetal echocardiography: accuracy and limitations in a population at high and low risk for heart defects. *Am. J. Obstet. Gynecol.*, **166**, 1473–81

16. Copel, J. A., Pilu, G., Green, J., Hobbins, J. C. and Kleinman, C. S. (1987). Fetal echocardiographic screening for congenital heart disease: the importance of the four-chamber view. *Am. J. Obstet. Gynecol.*, **157**, 648–55

17. Cullen, S., Sharland, G. K., Allan, L. D. and Sullivan, I. D. (1992). Potential impact of population screening for prenatal diagnosis of congenital heart disease. *Arch. Dis. Child.*, **67**, 775–8

18. Davis, G. K., Farquhar, C. M., Allan, L. D., Crawford, D. C. and Chapman, M. G. (1990). Structural cardiac abnormalities in the fetus: reliability of prenatal diagnosis and outcome. *Br. J. Obstet. Gynaecol.*, **97**, 27–31

19. DeVore, G. R. (1985). The prenatal diagnosis of congenital heart disease – a practical approach for the fetal sonographer. *J. Clin. Ultrasound*, **13**, 229–45

20. Fermont, L., deGeeter, B., Aubry, M. C., Kachaner, J. and Sidi, D. (1985). A close collaboration between obstetricians and pediatric cardiologists allows antenatal detection of severe cardiac malformations by two-dimensional echocardiography. In Doyle, E. F., Engle, M. A., Gersony, W. M., Rashkind, W. J. and Talner, N. S. (eds.) *Pediatric Cardiology, Proceedings of the 2nd World Congress*, pp. 34–7. (New York: Springer)

21. Hegge, F. N., Lees, M. H. and Watson, P. T. (1987). Utility of a screening examination of the fetal cardiac position and four chambers during obstetric sonography. *J. Reprod. Med.*, **32**, 353–8

22. Stewart, P. A., Wladimiroff, J. W., Reuss, A. and Sachs, E. S. (1987). Fetal echocardiography: a review of six years experience. *Fetal Ther.*, **2**, 222–31

23. Allan, L. D. (1989). Diagnosis of fetal cardiac abnormalities. *Arch. Dis. Child.*, **64**, 964–8

24. Cullen, S., Sharland, G. K., Allan, L. D. and Sullivan, I. D. (1992). Potential impact of population screening for prenatal diagnosis of congenital heart disease. *Arch. Dis. Child.*, **67**, 775–8

25. Greenwood, R. D., Rosenthal, A., Parisi, L., Fyler, D. C. and Nadas, A. S. (1975). Extracardiac abnormalities in infants with congenital heart disease. *Pediatrics*, **55**, 485

26. Wladimiroff, J. W., Stewart, P. A., Sachs, E. S. and Niermeijer, M. F. (1985). Prenatal diagnosis and management of congenital heart defect: significance of associated fetal anomalies and prenatal chromosome studies. *Am. J. Med. Genet.*, **21**, 285–90

27. Kleinman, C. S., Copel, J. A., Weinstein, E. M., Santulli, T. V. Jr and Hobbins, J. C. (1985). Treatment of fetal supraventricular tachyarrhythmias. *J. Clin. Ultrasound*, **13**, 265–73

28. Polak, P. E., Stewart, P. A. and Hess, J. (1989). Complete atrioventricular dissociation and His bundle tachycardia in a newborn: problems in prenatal diagnosis and postnatal management. *Int. J. Cardiol.*, **22**, 269–71

29. Stewart, P. A. and Wladimiroff, J. W. (1987). Cardiac tachyarrhythmia in the fetus: diagnosis, treatment and prognosis. *Fetal Ther.*, **2**, 7–16

30. Achiron, R., Glaser, J., Gelernter, I., Hegesh, J. and Yagel, S. (1992). Extended fetal echocardiographic examination for detecting cardiac malformations in low risk pregnancies. *Br. Med. J.*, **304**, 671–4

31. Rustico, M. A., Benettoni, A., D'Ottavio, G. *et al.* (1990). Fetal echocardiography: the role of the screening procedure. *Eur. J. Obstet. Gynecol. Reprod. Biol.*, **36**, 19–25

32. Sharland, G. K. and Allan, L. D. (1992). Screening for congenital heart disease prenatally. Results of a 2 1/2-year study in the South East Thames Region. *Br. J. Obstet. Gynaecol.*, **99**, 220–5

33. Tegnander, E., Eik-Nes, S. H. and Linker, D. (1991). Four-chamber view of the fetal heart – can more heart defects be detected on the routine scan? *6th World Congress on Ultrasound*, World Federation for Ultrasound in Medicine and Biology, Copenhagen, 1991

34. Vergani, P., Mariani, S., Ghidini, A., Schiavina, R., Cavallone, M., Locatelli, A., Strobelt, N. and Cerruti, P. (1992). Screening for congenital heart disease with the 4-chamber view of the fetal heart. *Am. J. Obstet. Gynecol.*, **167**, 1000–3

35. Buskens, E., Grobbee, D. E., Hess, J. and Wladimiroff, J. W. (1995). Prenatal screening for congenital heart disease; prospects and problems. *Eur. J. Obstet. Gynecol. Reprod. Biol.*, **60**, 5–11

36. Exalto, N. (1993). Guidelines on obstetric ultrasound examination and reporting. (Richtlijnen voor echoscopisch onderzoek en verslaglegging tijdens de zwangerschap.) Note on ultrasound in obstetrics and gynecology. (Nota echoscopie gynaecology/verloskunde.) *Werkgroep Echoscopie, NVOG en Sectie Obstetrie en Gynaecologie, NVUGB*, 11–14

37. Gert, A. L. and Moise, A. A. (1990). Fetal circulation and changes occurring at birth. In Garson, A., Bricker, J. T. and McNamara, D. G. (eds.) *The Science and Practice of Pediatric Cardiology*, pp. 280–8. (Malvern, Pennsylvania: Lea & Febiger)

38. Colton, T. (1974). *Statistics in Medicine.* (Boston, Massachusetts: Little, Brown and Co.)

39. Hoffman, J. I. (1990). Congenital heart disease: incidence and inheritance. *Pediatr. Clin. North Am.*, **37**, 25–43

40. Allan, L. D., Sharland, G. and Tynan, M. J. (1989). The natural history of the hypoplastic left heart syndrome. *Int. J. Cardiol.*, **25**, 341–3

41. Ewigman, B. G., Crane, J. P., Frigoletto, F. D., Lefevre, M. L., Bain, R. P. and Mcnellis, D. (1993). Effect of prenatal ultrasound screening on perinatal outcome. *N. Engl. J. Med.*, **329**, 21–7

42. Luck, C. A. (1992). Value of routine ultrasound scanning at 19 weeks: a four year study of 8849 deliveries. *Br. Med. J.*, **304**, 1474–8

43. Lys, F., De Wals, P., Borlee-Grimee, I., Billiet, A., Vincotte-Mols, M. and Levi, S. (1989). Evaluation of routine ultrasound examination for the prenatal diagnosis of malformation. *Eur. J. Obstet. Gynecol. Reprod. Biol.*, **30**, 101–19

44. Members of the Joint Study Group on Fetal Abnormalities (1989). Recognition and management of fetal abnormalities. *Arch. Dis. Child.*, **64**, 971–6

45. Wyllie, J., Wren, C. and Hunter, S. (1994). Screening for fetal cardiac malformations. *Br. Heart J.*, **71**, 20–7

46. Rosendahl, H. and Kivenen, S. (1989). Antenatal detection of congenital malformations by routine ultrasonography. *Obstet. Gynecol.*, **73**, 947–51

47. Achiron, R., Glaser, J., Gelernter, I., Hegesh, J. and Yagel, S. (1992). Extended fetal echocardiographic examination for detecting cardiac malformations in low risk pregnancies. *Br. Med. J.*, **304**, 671–4

48. Tenander, E., Eik-Nes, S. H. and Linker, D. (1991). Four-chamber view of the fetal heart – can more heart defects be detected on the routine scan? *6th World Congress in Ultrasound*, WFUMB, Copenhagen, 1991 (abstract)

49. Ursell, P. C., Byrne, J. M. and Strobino, B. A. (1985). Significance of cardiac defects in the developing fetus: a study of spontaneous abortuses. *Circulation*, **72**, 1232–6

50. Chinn, A., Fitzsimmons, J., Shepard, T. H. and Fantel, A. G. (1989). Congenital heart disease among spontaneous abortuses and stillborn fetuses: prevalence and associations. *Teratology*, **40**, 475–82

51. Buskens, E., Steyerberg, E. W., Hess, J., Wladimiroff, J. W. and Grobbee, D. E. (1995). Routine screening for congenital heart disease; what can be expected? A decision analytic approach. *Am. J. Publ. Health*, in press

# Ultrasonic evaluation of fetal cardiac function

8

*G. Rizzo, D. Arduini, A. Capponi and C. Romanini*

## INTRODUCTION

The intrauterine environment has limited in the past the possibility of studying the circulation in the human fetus and much of the understanding and present knowledge of fetal hemodynamics are derived from animal studies[1,2]. Moreover, during the last few years, technological advances in ultrasound have made it possible to study the human fetal heart. In particular, the advent of pulsed and color Doppler techniques has allowed the non-invasive examination of fetal cardiovascular pathophysiology, thus enabling hemodynamic studies on the fetus, both under normal and abnormal conditions.

This chapter will outline the principles of Doppler ultrasonography and its practical uses in the study of fetal cardiac function, and discuss its current and possible future applications.

## TECHNIQUE

### General principles

The parameters used to describe fetal cardiac velocity waveforms differ from those used in fetal peripheral vessels. In this latter situation, indices such as pulsatility index, resistance index or S/D ratio are used. These indices are derived from relative ratios between systolic, diastolic and mean velocity and are therefore independent from the absolute velocity values and from the angle of insonation between the Doppler beam and the direction of the blood flow[3].

Besides, at cardiac level all the measurements represent absolute values. Measurements of absolute flow velocities require knowledge of the angle of insonation which may be difficult to obtain with accuracy. The error in the estimation of the absolute velocity resulting from the uncertainty of angle measurement is strongly dependent on the magnitude of the angle itself. For angles less than about 20°, the error will be reduced to practical insignificance. For larger angles, the cosine term in the Doppler equation changes the small uncertainty in the measurement of the angle to a large error in velocity equations[3]. As a consequence, recordings should always be obtained keeping the Doppler beam as parallel to the bloodstream as possible and all the recordings with an estimated angle greater than 20° should be rejected.

Color Doppler may solve many of these problems by showing the flow direction in real time, allowing proper alignment of the Doppler beam in the direction of the blood flow. To record velocity waveforms, pulsed Doppler is generally preferred to continuous wave Doppler because of its range resolution. During recordings, the sample volume is placed immediately distal to the location to be investigated (e.g. distal to the aortic semilunar valves to record left ventricle outflow). However, in conditions of particularly high velocities (e.g. in the ductus arteriosus), continuous Doppler may be useful because it avoids the aliasing effect.

### Parameters measured

The parameters most commonly used to describe the cardiac velocity waveforms are the following:

(1) The *peak velocity* (PV) expressed as the maximum velocity at a given moment (e.g. systole, diastole) on the Doppler spectrum;

(2) The *time to peak velocity* (TPV) or acceleration time expressed by the time interval between the onset of the waveform and its peak; and

(3) The *time velocity integral* (TVI) calculated by planimetering the area underneath the Doppler spectrum.

It is possible also to calculate *absolute cardiac flow* from both atrioventricular valve and outflow tracts by multiplying the TVI by the valve area by the fetal heart rate. These measurements are particularly prone to errors, mainly due to inaccuracies in valve area. Area is derived from the valve diameter which is near the limits of ultrasound resolution and is then squared in its calculation, thus amplifying potential errors. However, they can be used properly in longitudinal studies at short time intervals in which the valve dimensions are assumed to remain constant. Furthermore, it is also possible to calculate accurately the relative ratio between the right and left cardiac outputs (RCO/LCO) avoiding measurements of cardiac valve size as the relative dimensions of aorta and pulmonary valves remain constant throughout gestation in the absence of cardiac structural disease[4].

## Site of recordings, velocity waveform characteristics and their significance

In the human, fetus blood flow velocity waveforms might be recorded at all cardiac levels including venous return, foramen ovale, atrioventricular valves, outflow tract and ductus arteriosus. Various factors affect the morphology of the velocity waveforms from different districts. Among these are preload[5,6], afterload[6,7], myocardial contractility[8], ventricular compliance[9] and fetal heart rate[10]. The impossibility of obtaining simultaneous recordings of pressure and volume does not allow full differentiation between these factors in the human fetus. However, as each parameter and site of recording are more specifically affected by one of these fac-

tors, it is possible to elucidate indirectly the underlying pathophysiology by performing measurements at various cardiac levels.

### Venous circulation

Blood flow velocity waveforms may be recorded from superior and inferior vena cava, ductus venosus, hepatic veins and pulmonary veins, as well as from the umbilical vein. The vascular district studied in more detail is the inferior vena cava. The inferior vena cava velocity waveforms, recorded from the segment of the vessel just distal to the entrance of the ductus venosus[11] (Color plate K), are characterized by a triphasic profile with a first forward wave concomitant with ventricular systole, a second forward wave of smaller dimensions occurring with early diastole and a third wave with reverse flow during atrial contraction[12] (Figure 1). Several indices have been suggested to analyze the inferior vena cava waveforms but the most frequently used is the percentage reverse flow quantified as the percentage of TVI during atrial contraction (reverse flow) with respect to total forward TVI (first and second waves)[12]. This index is considered to be related to the pressure gradient present between the right atrium and the right ventricle during end diastole, which is a

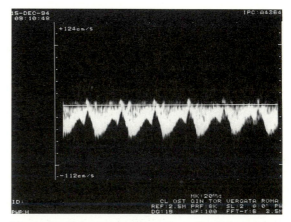

**Figure 1** Velocity waveforms from the inferior vena cava in a normal fetus at 36 weeks of gestation. Note the small amount of reverse flow during atrial contraction (upper panel)

function of both ventricular compliance and ventricular end-diastolic pressure[13].

The ductus venosus may be demonatrated in a transverse cross-section of the upper fetal abdomen at the level of its origin from the umbilical vein. The color is then superimposed and the pulsed Doppler sample volume is placed just above its inlet (close to the umbilical vein) at the point of maximum flow velocity as expressed by color brightness. Ductus venosus flow velocity waveforms exhibit a biphasic pattern with a first peak concomitant with systole (S), a second peak concomitant with diastole (D) and a nadir during atrial contraction (A) (Figure 2). Among the indices suggested to quantify velocity waveforms from the ductus venosus, the ratio between S peak velocity to A peak velocity (S/A) proved to be an angle-independent parameter that efficiently described ductus venosus hemodynamics[14].

The morphology of the velocity waveforms from hepatic veins is similar to that of the inferior vena cava. There is a scarcity of reports on the use of these vessels in the human fetus and, from the data available, it may be argued that the analysis of these vessels may have the same significance as that of the inferior vena cava.

Pulmonary vein velocity waveforms may be recorded at the level of their entrance in the left atrium. Their morphology is similar to that of the ductus venosus and is characterized by positive velocities during atrial contraction (Figure 3). The striking variations in the morphology of the velocity waveforms between the inferior vena cava and the pulmonary vein are of interest and reflect the different hemodynamic conditions occurring in the systemic and pulmonary circulations during intrauterine life.

Umbilical venous blood flow is usually continuous (Figure 4). However, in the presence of a relevant amount of reverse flow in the inferior vena cava during atrial contraction, pulsations with heart rate in umbilical venous flow have been noted. In normal pregnancies, these pulsations occur only before the 12th week of gestation and they are secondary to the stiffness of the ventricles present at this gestational age causing a high percentage of reverse

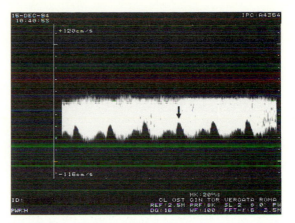

**Figure 2** Velocity waveforms from the ductus venosus in a normal fetus at 34 weeks of gestation. Note the presence of forward flow during atrial contraction (arrow)

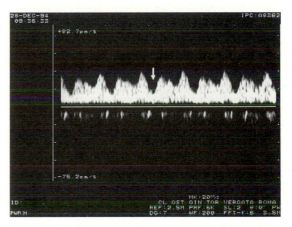

**Figure 3** Velocity waveforms from the left pulmonary vein in a normal fetus at 36 weeks of gestation. Note the presence of forward flow during atrial contraction (arrow)

flow in the inferior vena cava[15]. Later in gestation, the presence of pulsations in the umbilical vein expresses severe cardiac compromise.

### Atrioventricular valves

Flow velocity waveforms at the level of mitral and tricuspid valves are recorded from the apical four-chamber view of the fetal heart and are characterized by two diastolic peaks corresponding to early ventricular filling (E wave) and to active ventricular filling during atrial contraction (A wave) (Color plate L). The ratio between E and A waves (E/A) is a widely accepted index of ventricular diastolic function and is an expression of both the cardiac compliance and preload conditions[5,16] (Figure 5).

### Outflow tracts

Flow velocity waveforms from aorta and pulmonary artery are recorded from the five-chamber (Color plate M) and short-axis (Color plate N) views of the fetal heart, respectively. PV and TPV are the most commonly used indices. The former is influenced by several factors including valve size, myocardial contractility and afterload[6,7] while the latter is believed to be secondary to the mean arterial pressure[17].

### Pulmonary vessels

Velocity waveforms may be recorded from the right and left pulmonary arteries or from peripheral vessels within the lung. The morphology of the waveforms is different according to the site of sampling and their analysis may be used to study normal development of the lung circulation (Figures 6 and 7; Color plate O).

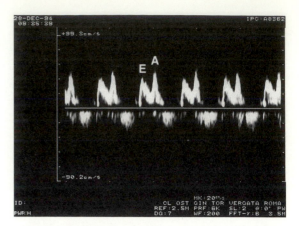

**Figure 5** Velocity waveforms from the mitral valve in a normal fetus at 34 weeks of gestation. The E/A ratio is equal to 0.81

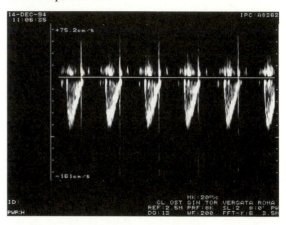

**Figure 6** Velocity waveforms from the main pulmonary artery in a normal fetus at 34 weeks of gestation

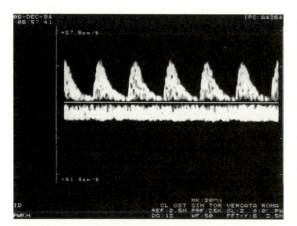

**Figure 4** Velocity waveforms from the umbilical artery and vein in a normal fetus at 16 weeks of gestation. Note the presence of continuous flow in the umbilical vein

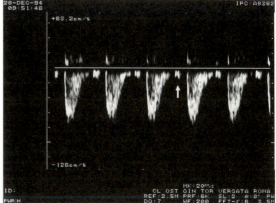

**Figure 7** Velocity waveforms from the right pulmonary artery in a normal fetus at 34 weeks of gestation. Note the presence of protodiastolic notch (arrow)

*Ductus arteriosus*

Ductal velocity waveforms are recorded from a short-axis view showing the ductal arch and are characterized by a continuous forward flow through the entire cardiac cycle[18]. The parameters most commonly analyzed are the PV during systole or, similarly to peripheral vessels, the pulsatility index (PI = [systolic velocity − diastolic velocity]/mean velocity)[19,20].

## Reproducibility

A major concern in obtaining absolute measurements of velocities of flow is their reproducibility. In order to obtain reliable recordings, it is particularly important to minimize the angle of insonation as mentioned above, to verify in real time and color flow imaging the correct position of the sample volume before and after each Doppler recording, and to limit the recordings to periods of fetal rest and apnea, as behavioral states greatly influence the recordings[20]. Under these conditions, it is necessary to select a series (in our center, 10) of consecutive velocity waveforms characterized by uniform morphology and high signal/noise ratio before performing the measurements. Using this technique of recording and analysis, we managed to obtain a coefficient of variation below 10% for all the echocardiographic indices with the exception of the valve dimensions. These results are in agreement with those reported by other centers (Groenenberg and co-workers[21], coefficient of variation < 7%; Al-Ghazali and co-workers[22], coefficient of variation < 7.6%; Reed and co-workers[23], maximal variation < 10%).

## NORMAL RANGES OF CARDIAC DOPPLER INDICES

The advent of transvaginal color Doppler equipment has allowed flow velocity waveforms to be recorded from 11 weeks of gestation onwards[24]. Marked changes occur at all cardiac levels from this gestational age up to 20 weeks. The percentage reverse flow in the inferior vena cava significantly decreases[14,25], the E/A ratio at both atrioventricular levels dramatically increases[24,25],

PV and TVI values in outflow tracts increase and this is particularly evident at the level of the pulmonary valve[24]. These changes suggest a rapid development of ventricular compliance (that may explain the decrease of inferior vena cava reverse flow and the increase of E/A) and a shift of cardiac output toward the right ventricle probably secondary to decreased right ventricle afterload due to the fall of placental resistance.

After 20 weeks of gestation, there is a further but less evident decrease of inferior vena cava reverse flow[26] associated with a significant decrease of the S/A ratio from the ductus venosus[14].

At the level of the atrioventricular valves, the E/A ratios increase[27,28], while PV values linearly increase at the level of both pulmonary and aortic valves[29]. Small changes are present in TPV values during gestation[30]. TPV values at the level of the pulmonary valve are lower than at aortic level, suggesting a slightly higher blood pressure in the pulmonary artery than in the ascending aorta[31]. Quantitative measurements have shown that the right cardiac output (RCO) is higher than the left cardiac output (LCO) and that from 20 weeks onwards the RCO/LCO ratio remains constant with a mean value of 1.3[32,33]. This value is lower than that reported in fetal sheep (RCO/LCO = 1.8) and this difference may be explained by the higher brain weight in humans which increases the left cardiac output[34].

Ductal PV increases linearly with gestation and its values represent the highest velocity in the fetal circulation under normal conditions[18,19]. Values of systolic velocity above 140 cm/s in conjunction with a diastolic velocity > 35 cm/s are considered to be an expression of ductal constriction[18].

## CARDIAC DOPPLER FINDINGS IN ABNORMAL GESTATIONS

### Growth-retarded fetuses

Intrauterine growth-retarded (IUGR) fetuses secondary to uteroplacental insufficiency are characterized by selective changes of peripheral vascular resistances (i.e. the so-called brain-sparing effect) that influence cardiac hemodynamics[35]. Secondary to the brain-sparing condition, selective modifications occur in cardiac afterload with a decreased left ventricle afterload due to cerebral vasodilatation and an increased right ventricle afterload as a result of the systemic vasoconstriction. Furthermore, hypoxemia might impair myocardial contractility while polycythemia might alter blood viscosity and therefore preload.

As a consequence, IUGR fetuses show impaired ventricular filling properties with a lower E/A ratio at the level of the atrioventricular valves[28], lower PV in aorta and pulmonary arteries[36], increased aortic and decreased pulmonary TPV[30] and a relative increase of LCO associated with decreased RCO[22]. These hemodynamic intracardiac changes are compatible with a preferential shift of cardiac output in favor of the left ventricle, leading to improved perfusion to the brain. Thus, in the first stages of the disease, the supply of substrates and oxygen can be maintained at near normal levels despite an absolute reduction of placental transfer.

Longitudinal studies of progressively deteriorating IUGR fetuses have allowed the elucidation of the natural history of these hemodynamic modifications during uteroplacental insufficiency[26,36]. Such studies have shown that both TPV in the aorta and pulmonary arteries and the ratios between right and left ventricle outputs remain stable during serial recordings. These findings are consistent with the absence of other significant changes in outflow resistances (a parameter inversely related to TPV values) and with cardiac output redistribution after the establishment of the brain-sparing mechanism[36]. However, in deteriorating IUGR fetuses, PV and cardiac output gradually decline, suggesting a progressive decline in cardiac function[36] (Color plate P). As a consequence cardiac filling may be impaired. Studies in the fetal venous circulation[26] have demonstrated that an increase of inferior vena cava reverse flow during atrial contraction occurs with progressive fetal deterioration, suggesting a higher pressure gradient in the right atrium (Color plate Q). The next step of the disease is exten-sion of abnormal reversal of blood velocities in the inferior vena cava to the ductus venosus, inducing an increase of the S/A ratio mainly due to a reduction of the A component of the velocity waveforms[14] (Color plate R). Finally, the high venous pressure induces a reduction of velocity at end diastole in the umbilical vein causing typical end-diastolic pulsations[37] (Color plate S). The development of these pulsations is close to the onset of fetal heart rate anomalies and is frequently associated with acidemia at birth[37,38].

## Fetuses of diabetic mothers

Infants of diabetic mothers have long been recognized to be at risk of developing hypertrophic cardiomyopathy[39]. This disease is characterized by a thickening of the interventricular septum and ventricular free walls and by systolic and diastolic dysfunction of the neonatal heart, which may result in congestive heart failure in the immediate postnatal period[40]. Echocardiographic studies of the fetal heart have demonstrated that hypertrophic cardiomyopathy may be present prenatally and develop progressively with fetal growth.

M-mode studies in fetuses of insulin-dependent diabetic mothers have shown an increased thickness of ventricular walls that is particularly evident at the level of interventricular septum[41–43]. The increased cardiac size does not merely reflect the larger size of fetuses of diabetic mothers (i.e. macrosomia), but represents a selective organomegaly. Indeed, controlling cardiac size for fetal abdominal circumference or biparietal diameter, biometric parameters closely related to fetal weight, showed increased wall thickness in fetuses of diabetic mothers irrespective of fetal size[41,42].

Longitudinal echocardiographic studies have allowed the natural history of the development of fetal hypertrophic cardiomyopathy to be elucidated. Fetuses of diabetic mothers showed an accelerated increase of cardiac size and the growth curves differ from those of normal fetuses[44]. Although the cardiac walls are already thicker than in normal fetuses at 20 weeks of gestation, the accelerated increase of cardiac size is mainly evident during the late second trimester[44]. The cause of a higher growth rate of cardiac size during the late second trimester is unclear. Because no differences were present in the metabolic control, it has been speculated that there may be a different degree of sensitivity of the fetal myocardium to factors accelerating its growth. This hypothesis is supported by the data of Thorsson and Hinz[45] showing a reduction from fetus to adult in the number and affinity of insulin receptors.

Echocardiographic studies[41,44] have shown that the increase of cardiac wall thickness influences fetal cardiac function.

Fetuses of diabetic mothers show lower E/A ratios at the level of both atrioventricular valves when compared to normal fetuses[44] (Figure 8). Longitudinal studies have shown that these changes are already present in early gestation and that a delayed development of diastolic function occurs, with a slower rate of change of E/A ratios, during pregnancy[44].

The low E/A values might be explained by an impaired development of ventricular compliance in fetuses of diabetic mothers secondary to cardiac wall thickening. This is consistent with the significant relationship existing between both interventricular septum and lateral ventricular wall thickness and the severity of the impairment of E/A values[41].

Moreover, the E/A ratio is also influenced by the preload as reported above. Polycythemia is frequently present at birth in infants of diabetic mothers[46]. This condition increases blood viscosity which may reduce preload, and thus potentially affects the E/A ratio also during intrauterine life. This hypothesis is supported by recent data showing a significant relationship between fetal hematocrit and the E/A values after controlling values for cardiac thickness and fetal heart rate[47], thus suggesting a significant role of fetal blood viscosity on cardiac diastolic function.

Peak velocities at the level of aortic and pulmonary outflow tracts were significantly higher in fetuses of diabetic mothers than in normal fetuses[41]. Increased PV could be secondary to reduced outflow tract dimensions, decreased afterload, increased cardiac contractility, or in-

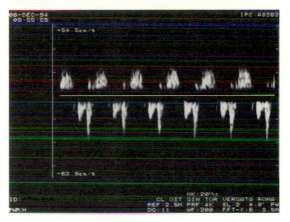

**Figure 8** Velocity waveforms from the mitral valve in a fetus of a diabetic mother at 34 weeks of gestation. The E/A ratio is equal to 0.51 (normal mean for gestation 0.77). Note the difference from Figure 5

creased flow volume. Differentiation between these factors is difficult in the human fetus. An obstruction of the left ventricular outflow tract due to hypertrophy of the septal musculature resulting in an increase in aortic PV has been described in infants of diabetic mothers[48]. However, in this condition, the obstruction is usually limited to the left ventricular outflow tract and not affecting the right ventricle, thus not explaining the presence of a concomitant increase of pulmonary PV. Similarly, a decrease in afterload seems unlikely on the basis of a lack of difference between control fetuses and fetuses of diabetic mothers in time to peak velocity. An increased contractility is compatible with postnatal studies, showing a systolic ventricular contractile function above normal in infants of diabetic mothers[49]. Finally, the higher values of the peak velocity present in fetuses of diabetic mothers may be explained on the basis of increased intracardiac flow volume secondary to a relatively larger fetal size of such fetuses since cardiac output is a function of fetal weight.

These abnormalities in cardiac hemodynamics also impair the venous circulation. We have recently shown that the percentage reverse flow in the inferior vena cava is increased in fetuses of diabetic mothers. Furthermore, fetuses with a percentage reverse flow in the inferior vena cava above 2 SDs from the expected mean for gestation showed at birth a lower pH in the umbilical artery, an increased hematocrit and a higher morbidity[50]. Besides, no variations were evidenced in fetal peripheral vessels.

Based on these observations, we speculated that the mechanisms inducing fetal distress are different in fetuses of diabetic mothers compared with IUGR fetuses. In the former group, the development of hypertrophic cardiomyopathy plays a pivotal role in the genesis of fetal distress, while in the latter group the changes in cardiac function are secondary to modification in peripheral resistances.

After birth, the hypertrophic changes of the myocardium regress to normal over a period of several months and are usually no longer present at 1 year of age[40,49]. There is no account, however, whether these perinatal modifications may affect cardiac function during adult life. Moreover, significant changes occur during the transitional circulation. In normal fetuses, the E/A ratios at the level of both atrioventricular valves significantly increase during the first days of life and the E wave is usually higher than the A wave resulting in an E/A ratio higher than 1[51]. In newborns of diabetic mothers, no changes of E/A ratio occur during the first 5 days of life and its value remains lower than 1[51]. These anomalies might explain the relatively high incidence of transitory tachypnea and pulmonary edema present in those infants immediately after birth[16].

## Fetal anemia

Red cell isoimmunization results in a progressive destruction of fetal red cells leading to fetal anemia. Furthermore, intravascular fetal blood transfusion by cordocentesis represents the standard treatment of fetal anemia and this procedure leads to rapid injection of large amount of blood with respect to fetoplacental volume.

Doppler echocardiography has made it possible to elucidate the hemodynamic response of the human fetus to anemia and its rapid correction[52,53].

Before transfusion (in a condition of anemia), the left and right cardiac outputs are significantly higher than normal and a significant relationship is present between the severity of fetal anemia and cardiac output[52,53]. As a consequence of the high volume flow, PV at outflow tract level is also increased[52]. Furthermore, the E/A ratio at both atrioventricular valves is increased[53]. Venous flow is similarly affected with an increase of peak velocities in the ductus venosus[54].

The fetal cardiac output is increased, presumably to maintain adequate oxygen delivery to organs. Although the mechanisms causing the increase of cardiac output are still unclear, two main factors have been suggested[55]: first, decreased blood viscosity leading to increased venous return and cardiac preload, and second, peripheral vasodilatation due to a fall in blood oxygen content and therefore reduced cardiac afterload. The first mechanism is supported by the high E/A values from atrioventricular valves present in anemic fetuses.

Besides there is no evidence for a redistribution of cardiac output similar to that described in hypoxic IUGR fetuses (brain-sparing effect) since the RCO/LCO ratio is normal in anemic fetuses[53]. This is in agreement with the normal values of PI present in fetal peripheral vessels of anemic fetuses[55]. These findings suggest that, in red cell isoimmunization, the changes in fetal cardiac function are mainly related to the low blood viscosity leading to a hyperdynamic situation.

After intravascular transfusion, there is a significant temporary fall in right and left cardiac outputs[52,53] associated with increased E/A ratios[53] (Color plate T). The latter changes may be related to the increased preload secondary to the relatively large amount of blood transfused.

The decrease in cardiac output may be secondary to four different factors (heart rate, preload, myocardial contractility, or afterload). The first factor may be excluded as cardiac output also decreases in the absence of any significant changes in fetal heart rate[52]. Preload should be decreased to support the decrease of cardiac output, but the high E/A values suggest an increase of preload rather than a decrease[53]. Similarly, an impaired myocardial contractility seems unlikely on the basis of the velocity waveforms in aorta and pulmonary artery[53]. Therefore, an increase in cardiac afterload seems to offer the best explanation for the decrease in cardiac output[53]. This hypothesis is consistent with experimental animal studies showing after transfusion a marked increase in mean arterial pressure and therefore in cardiac afterload[57].

It is noteworthy that the fall of cardiac output in the human fetus is significantly related to the amount of expansion of the fetoplacental volume[53]. Moreover, within 2 hours of transfusion, all the echocardiographic parameters return towards the normal range suggesting a rapid recovery of the fetal circulation to volume expansion[53].

## Discordant twins

Twin pregnancies have a high rate of perinatal complications which are particularly evident in pairs with discordant growth[58]. Studies limited to umbilical artery have provided conflicting results in twins about whether discordant size is associated with discordant Doppler indices[59–62]. These discrepancies may be explained on the basis of the different classification criteria followed.

In a recent study we carefully selected two groups of twin pregnancies with discordant growth classified with rigid criteria[63]. In the first group, the etiology is malnutrition of one twin due to placental insufficiency limited to one placenta. Indeed, criteria of inclusion were presence of dichorionic placentas, thus virtually excluding the possibility of blood shunts between fetuses, absence of chromosomal and structural anomalies, excluding intrinsic causes of the growth defect, and an indication for delivery based on the presence of late decelerations suggestive of fetal hypoxemia of the smaller twin. In the larger twin, serial recordings showed the absence of any differences with respect to normal singleton pregnancies in all the vessels investigated, thus suggesting normal placental and fetal hemodynamics. On the other hand, the smaller twin showed progressive changes of Doppler indices similar to those described earlier in singleton growth-retarded fetuses secondary to placental insufficiency. As a consequence of these hemodynamic changes,

the absolute values of the Doppler indices in the smaller twin or the delta values between the smaller and the larger twin may serve as a tool for fetal surveillance or prediction of fetal distress similar to what happens in singleton pregnancies. This confirms previous studies showing how a high differential value between the pulsatility indices in the umbilical arteries can predict low birth weight and adverse perinatal outcome in twin pregnancies[59,60]. The combined study of several vascular districts may improve the diagnostic efficacy of Doppler ultrasonography.

The second group of twin pregnancies studied was secondary to twin-to-twin transfusion syndrome. The classic pathophysiologic background of this syndrome is a shift of blood volume from one donor twin to the recipient twin[64]. As a result of the transfusions, the donor twin becomes anemic, decreases its growth rate, and develops oligohydramnios as a consequence of oliguria, while the recipient twin becomes polycythemic and plethoric and as a result of the volume overload may develop polyhydramnios, cardiomegaly, cardiac insufficiency and hydrops[64]. However, this concept has been questioned recently by data obtained at cordocentesis showing small differences in cord hemoglobin between fetuses with classical signs of twin-to-twin transfusion syndrome[65]. This suggests that the mechanism generating this syndrome is more complex than mere shifts of blood volume that probably become massive only at a late stage of the disease. Our serial recordings obtained in this second group of twin fetuses support this concept by showing changes of Doppler indices only at the time of the last recording, close to the delivery due to fetal distress in most of the cases. These changes are present at cardiac and venous level and are consistent with a condition of anemia (increased PV at outflow tract and decreased percentage reverse flow in inferior vena cava) in the smaller twin and of massive blood transfusion (decreased PV at outflow tract, increased percentage reverse flow in the inferior vena cava and umbilical vein pulsations) in the larger twin. Indeed, these Doppler patterns are similar to those described before and immediately after intravascular blood transfusion. The absence of differences in PI values from fetal vessels also close to delivery is not surprising as these indices are minimally affected by fetal anemia or polycythemia[56] and this confirms previous reports limited to the umbilical artery[60].

The absence of evident changes of cardiac and venous Doppler indices in the weeks preceding delivery, despite the growth discordance between twins and the presence of oligohydramnios and polyhydramnios, suggests a different pathophysiological mechanism at an early stage of the syndrome. It has been suggested that twin-to-twin transfusion syndrome may develop first as a consequence of placental insufficiency affecting the donor twin[65]. According to this hypothesis, placental insufficiency increases vascular resistance in the donor twin resulting in a preferential shunt, at a later stage of the disease, toward the recipient twin. Our data do not allow us to support this theory as we were unable to document in serial recordings any Doppler changes suggestive of placental insufficiency.

## CONCLUSION

Doppler ultrasound has enabled non-invasive studies of the fetal circulation under physiological and pathological conditions. These studies have demonstrated cardiovascular changes occurring in the human fetus in different clinical conditions. The knowledge from these data may prove useful in improving the diagnosis, monitoring and treatment of compromised fetuses.

# References

1. Edelstone, D. I. and Rudolph, A. M. (1979). Preferential streaming of ductus venosus blood to the brain and heart in fetal lambs. *Am. J. Physiol.*, **237**, H724–9

2. Rudolph, A. M. (1985). Distribution and regulation of blood flow in the fetal and neonatal lamb. *Circ. Res.*, **57**, 811–21

3. Burns, P. N. (1987). Doppler flow estimations in the fetal and maternal circulations: principles, techniques and some limitations. In Maulik, D. and McNellis, D. (Eds.) *Doppler Ultrasound Measurement of Maternal–Fetal Hemodynamics*, pp. 43–78. (Ithaca, New York: Perinatology Press)

4. Comstock, C. H., Riggs, T., Lee, W. and Kirk, J. (1991). Pulmonary to aorta diameter ratio in the normal and abnormal fetal heart. *Am. J. Obstet. Gynecol.*, **165**, 1038–43

5. Stottard, M. F., Pearson, A. C., Kern, M. J., Ratcliff, J., Mrosek, D. G. and Labovitz, A. J. (1989). Influence of alteration in preload of left ventricular diastolic filling as assessed by Doppler echocardiography in humans. *Circulation*, **79**, 1226–36

6. Gardin, J. M. (1989). Doppler measurements of aortic blood velocity and acceleration: load-independent indexes of left ventricular performance. *Am. J. Cardiol.*, **64**, 935–6

7. Bedotto, J. B., Eichorn, E. J. and Grayburn, P. A. (1989). Effects of left ventricular preload and afterload on ascendic aortic blood velocity and acceleration in coronaric artery disease. *Am. J. Cardiol.*, **64**, 856–9

8. Brownwall, E., Ross, J. and Sonnenblick, E. H. (1976). *Mechanism of Contraction in the Normal and Failing Heart.* 2nd edn., pp. 92–129. (Boston: Little Brown)

9. Takaneka, K., Dabestani, A., Gardin, J. M., Russel, D., Clark, S., Allfie, A. and Henry, W. L. (1986). Left ventricular filling in hypertrophic cardiomyopathy: a pulsed Doppler echocardiographic study. *J. Am. Coll. Cardiol.*, **7**, 1263–71

10. Kenny, J., Plappert, T., Doubilet, P., Saltzam, D. and St. John Sutton, M. G. (1987). Effects of heart rate on ventricular size, stroke volume and output in the normal human fetus: a prospective Doppler echocardiographic study. *Circulation*, **76**, 52–8

11. Rizzo, G., Caforio, L., Arduini, D. and Romanini, C. (1992). Effects of sampling site on inferior vena cava flow velocity waveforms. *J. Matern. Fetal Inv.*, **2**, 153–6

12. Reed, K. L., Appleton, C. P., Anderson, C. F., Shenker, L. and Sahn, D. J. (1990). Doppler studies of vena cava flows in human fetuses – insights into normal and abnormal cardiac physiology. *Circulation*, **81**, 498–505

13. Appleton, C. P., Hatle, L. K. and Popp, R. L. (1987). Superior vena cava and hepatic vein Doppler echocardiography in healthy adults. *J. Am. Coll. Cardiol.*, **10**, 1032–9

14. Rizzo, G., Capponi, A., Arduini, D. and Romanini, C. (1994). Ductus venosus velocity waveforms in appropriate and small for ges-tational age fetuses. *Early Hum. Dev.*, **37**, in press

15. Rizzo, G., Arduini, D. and Romanini, C. (1992). Pulsations in umbilical vein: a physiological finding in early pregnancy. *Am. J. Obstet. Gynecol.*, **167**, 675–7

16. Labovitz, A. J. and Pearson, C. (1987). Evaluation of left ventricular diastolic function: clinical relevance and recent Doppler echocardiographic insights. *Am. Heart J.*, **114**, 836–51

17. Kitabatake, A., Inoue, M., Asao, M., Masuyama, T., Tanouchi, J., Morita, T., Mishima, M., Uematsu, M., Shimazu, T., Hori, M. and Abe, H. (1983). Noninvasive evaluation of pulmonary hypertension by a pulsed Doppler technique. *Circulation*, **68**, 302–9

18. Huhta, J. C., Moise, K. J., Fisher, D. J., Sharif, D. F., Wasserstrum, N. and Martin, C. (1987). Detection and quantitation of constriction of the fetal ductus arteriosus by Doppler echocardiography. *Circulation*, **75**, 406–12

19. Van de Mooren, K., Barendregt, L. G. and Wladimiroff, J. (1991). Flow velocity waveforms in the human fetal ductus arteriosus during the normal second trimester of pregnancy. *Pediatr. Res.*, **30**, 487–90

20. Rizzo, G., Arduini, D., Valensise, H. and Romanini, C. (1990). Effects of behavioural states on cardiac output in the healthy human fetus at 36–38 weeks of gestation. *Early Hum. Dev.*, **23**, 109–15

21. Groenenberg, I. A. L., Hop, W. C. J. and Wladimiroff, J. W. (1991). Doppler flow velocity waveforms in the fetal cardiac outflow tract; reproducibility of waveform recording and analysis. *Ultrasound Med. Biol.*, **17**, 583–7

22. Al-Ghazali, W., Chita, S. K., Chapman, M. G. and Allan, L. D. (1989). Evidence of redistribution of cardiac output in asymmetrical growth retardation. *Br. J. Obstet. Gynaecol.*, **96**, 697–704

23. Reed, K. L., Meijboom, E. J., Sahn, D. J., Scagnelli, S. A., Valdes-Cruz, L. M. and Skenker, L. (1986). Cardiac Doppler flow velocities in human fetuses. *Circulation*, **73**, 41–56

24. Rizzo, G., Arduini, D. and Romanini, C. (1991). Fetal cardiac and extra-cardiac circulation in early gestation. *J. Matern. Fetal Invest.*, **1**, 73–8

25. Wladimiroff, J. W., Huisman, T. W. A., Stewart, P. A. and Stijnen, Th. (1992). Normal fetal Doppler inferior vena cava, transtricuspid and umbilical artery flow velocity waveforms between 11 and 16 weeks' gestation. *Am. J. Obstet. Gynecol.*, **166**, 46–9

26. Rizzo, G., Arduini, D. and Romanini, C. (1992). Inferior vena cava flow velocity waveforms in appropriate and small for gestational age fetuses. *Am. J. Obstet. Gynecol.*, **166**, 1271–80

27. Reed, K. L., Sahn, D. I., Scagnelli, S., Anderson, C. F. and Shenker, L. (1986). Doppler echocardiographic studies of diastolic function in the human fetal heart: changes during gestation. *J. Am. Coll. Cardiol.*, **8**, 391–5

28. Rizzo, G., Arduini, D., Romanini, C. and Mancuso, S. (1988). Doppler echocardiographic assessment of atrioventricular velocity waveforms in normal and small for gestational age fetuses. *Br. J. Obstet. Gynaecol.*, **95**, 65–9

29. Kenny, J. F., Plappert, T., Saltzman, D. H., Cartire, M., Zollars, L., Leatherman, G. F. and St John Sutton, M. G. (1986). Changes in intracardiac blood flow velocities and right and left ventricular stroke volumes with gestational age in the normal human fetus: a prospective Doppler echocardiographic study. *Circulation*, **74**, 1208–16

30. Rizzo, G., Arduini, D., Romanini, C. and Mancuso, S. (1990). Doppler echocardiographic evaluation of time to peak velocity in the aorta and pulmonary artery of small for gestational age fetuses. *Br. J. Obstet. Gynaecol.*, **97**, 603–7

31. Machado, M. V. L., Chita, S. C. and Allan, L. D. (1987). Acceleration time in the aorta and pulmonary artery measured by Doppler echocardiography in the midtrimester normal human fetus. *Br. Heart J.*, **58**, 15–18

32. Allan, L. D., Chita, S. K., Al-Ghazali, W., Crawford, D. C. and Tynan, M. (1987). Doppler echocardiographic evaluation of the normal human fetal heart. *Br. Heart J.*, **57**, 528–33

33. De Smedt, M. C. H., Visser, G. H. A. and Meijboom, E. J. (1987). Fetal cardiac output estimated by Doppler echocardiography during mid- and late gestation. *Am. J. Cardiol.*, **60**, 338–42

34. Rizzo, G. and Arduini, D. (1991). Cardiac output in anencephalic fetuses. *Gynecol. Obstet. Invest.*, **32**, 33–5

35. Peeters, L. L. H., Sheldon, R. F., Jones, M. D., Makowsky, E. I. and Meschia, G. (1979). Blood flow to fetal organ as a function of arterial oxygen content. *Am. J. Obstet. Gynecol.*, **135**, 637–46

36. Rizzo, G. and Arduini, D. (1991). Fetal cardiac function in intrauterine growth retardation. *Am. J. Obstet. Gynecol.*, **165**, 876–82

37. Arduini, D., Rizzo, G. and Romanini, C. (1993). The development of abnormal heart rate patterns after absent end diastolic velocity in umbilical artery: analysis of risk factors. *Am. J. Obstet. Gynecol.*, **168**, 43–9

38. Indick, J. H., Chen, V. and Reed, K. L. (1991). Association of umbilical venous with inferior vena cava blood flow velocities. *Obstet. Gynecol.*, **77**, 551–7

39. Gutgesell, H. P., Speer, M. E. and Rosenberg, H. S. (1980). Characterization of the cardiomyopathy in infants of diabetic mothers. *Circulation*, **61**, 441–50

40. Reller, M. D. and Kaplan, S. (1988). Hypertrophic cardiomyopathy in infants of diabetic mothers: an update. *Am. J. Perinatol.*, **5**, 353–8

41. Weber, H. S., Copel, J. A., Reece, A., Green, J. and Kleinman, C. S. (1991). Cardiac growth in fetuses of diabetic mothers with good metabolic control. *J. Pediatr.*, **118**, 103–7

42. Rizzo, G., Arduini, D. and Romanini, C. (1991). Cardiac function in fetuses of type I diabetic mothers. *Am. J. Obstet. Gynecol.*, **164**, 837–43

43. Vielle, J. C., Sivekoff, M., Hanson, R. and Fanaroff, A. A. (1992). Interventricular septal thickness in fetuses of diabetic mothers. *Obstet. Gynecol.*, **79**, 51–4

44. Rizzo, G., Arduini, D. and Romanini, C. (1992). Accelerated cardiac growth and abnormal cardiac flows in fetuses of type I diabetic mothers. *Obstet. Gynecol.*, **80**, 369–76

45. Thorsson, A. V. and Hintz, R. L. (1977). Insulin receptors in the newborn: increase in receptor affinity and number. *N. Engl. J. Med.*, **297**, 908–12

46. Widness, J., Susa, J. and Garcia, J. (1981). Increased erythropoiesis and elevated erythropoietin levels in infants born to diabetic mothers and in hyperinsulinemic rhesus fetuses. *J. Clin. Invest.*, **67**, 637–41

47. Rizzo, G., Pietropolli, A., Capponi, A., Cacciatore, C., Arduini, D. and Romanini, C. (1994). Analysis of factors affecting ventricular filling in fetuses of type I diabetic mothers. *J. Perinat. Med.*, **22**, 125–32

48. Gutgesell, H. P., Mullins, C. E., Gillette, P. C., Speer, M., Rudolph, A. J. and McNamara, D. G. (1976). Transient hypertrophic subaortic stenosis in infants of diabetic mothers. *J. Pediatr.*, **89**, 120–5

49. Mace, S., Hirschfeld, S. S., Riggs, T., Faranoff, A. A. and Mecketz, I. R. (1979). Echocardiographic abnormalities in infants of diabetic mothers. *J. Pediatr.*, **95**, 1013–19

50. Rizzo, G., Capponi, A., Rinaldo, D., Arduini, D. and Romanini, C. (1994). Inferior cava velocity waveforms predict neonatal complications in fetuses of insulin dependent diabetic mothers. *J. Matern. Fetal Invest.*, **4**, in press

51. Condoluci, C., Rizzo, G., Arduini, D. and Romanini, C. (1991). Transitional circulation in infants of diabetic mothers. In *6th Fetal Cardiology Symposium. Abstract Book*, p. 23. (Rome: CIC)

52. Moise, K. J., Mari, G., Fisher, D. J., Hutha, J. C., Cano, L. E. and Carpenter, R. J. (1990). Acute fetal hemodynamic alterations after intrauterine transfusion for treatment of severe red blood cell alloimmunization. *Am. J. Obstet. Gynecol.*, **163**, 776–84

53. Rizzo, G., Nicolaides, K. H., Arduini, D. and Campbell, S. (1990). Effects of intravascular fetal blood transfusion on fetal intracardiac Doppler velocity waveforms. *Am. J. Obstet. Gynecol.*, **163**, 1231–8

54. Oepkes, D., Vandenbussche, F. P., Van Bel, F. and Kanhai, H. H. H. (1993). Fetal ductus venosus blood flow velocities before and after transfusion in red-cell alloimmunized pregnancies. *Obstet. Gynecol.*, **82**, 237–41

55. Fumia, F. D., Edelstone, D. I. and Holzman, I. R. (1984). Blood flow and oxygen delivery as functions of fetal hematocrit. *Am. J. Obstet. Gynecol.*, **150**, 274–82

56. Bilardo, C. M., Nicolaides, K. H. and Campbell, S. (1989). Doppler studies in red cell isoimmunization. *Clin. Obstet. Gynecol.*, **32**, 719–27

57. Chestnut, D. H., Pollack, K. L., Weiner, C. P., Robillard, J. E., Thompson, C. S. and DeBruyn, C. S. (1989). Does furosemide alter the hemodynamic response to rapid intravascular transfusion of the anemic lamb fetus? *Am. J. Obstet. Gynecol.*, **161**, 1571–5

58. Ho, S. K. and Wu, P. K. (1975). Perinatal factors and neonatal morbidity in twin pregnancy. *Am. J. Obstet. Gynecol.*, **122**, 979–87

59. Farmakides, G., Schulman, H., Saldana, L. R., Bracero, L. A., Fleisher, A. and Rochelson, B. (1986). Surveillance of twin pregnancies with umbilical artery velocity waveforms. *Am. J. Obstet. Gynecol.*, **153**, 789–92

60. Giles, W. B., Trudinger, B. J. and Cook, C. M. (1985). Fetal umbilical artery velocity waveforms in twin pregnancies. *Br. J. Obstet. Gynaecol.*, **92**, 490–7

61. Pretorius, D. H., Machester, D., Barkin, S., Parker, S. and Nelson, T. R. (1988). Doppler ultrasound of twin–twin transfusion syndrome. *J. Ultrasound Med.*, **7**, 117–24

62. Giles, W. B., Trudinger, B. J., Cook, C. M. and Connelly, A. J. (1990). Doppler umbilical artery Doppler studies in the twin–twin transfusion syndrome. *Obstet. Gynecol.*, **76**, 1097–9

63. Rizzo, G., Arduini, D. and Romanini, C. (1994). Cardiac and extra-cardiac flows in discordant twins. *Am. J. Obstet. Gynecol.*, **170**, 1321–7

64. Blickstein, I. (1990). The twin–twin transfusion syndrome. *Obstet. Gynecol.*, **76**, 714–21

65. Saunders, N. J., Snijders, R. J. M. and Nicolaides, K. H. (1991). Twin–twin transfusion syndrome during the 2nd trimester is associated with small intertwin hemoglobin differences. *Fetal Diagn. Ther.*, **6**, 34–6

# Fetal arrhythmias

9

*J. A. Copel and C. S. Kleinman*

## INTRODUCTION

In this chapter we shall review the major fetal cardiac arrhythmias, their pathophysiology and clinical consequences, and their treatment. Fetal antiarrhythmic therapy must be based on an understanding of the underlying electrophysiology of the arrhythmia and on knowledge of feto–maternal pharmacology and the pharmacokinetics of antiarrhythmic drugs. Each antiarrhythmic agent carries the potential for significant toxicity to mothers and fetuses, so risks and benefits of fetal treatment should be carefully considered prior to any intervention. We will discuss selected treatment approaches, although space constraints preclude detailed discussion of the biochemistry of the drugs. An extensive review of the electrophysiology of fetal tachyarrhythmias and the drugs in common use for their treatment can be found in a number of recent publications[1,2].

## FETAL RHYTHM ANALYSIS

The electrocardiogram (ECG) is the ideal clinical tool for the analysis of arrhythmias, but is currently unavailable for use in the fetus other than by internal scalp electrodes in labor. Since most fetal arrhythmias require diagnosis before the onset of labor, other non–invasive approaches must be utilized. Echocardiographic techniques for fetal cardiac rhythm analysis include m-mode, pulsed Doppler and Doppler color flow encoded m-mode imaging.

In the absence of an electrocardiographic tracing providing information about electrical depolarization of the atria (P waves) and ventricles (QRS complexes), cardiac ultrasound can be used to detect mechanical events in the cardiac cycle. These represent the mechanical responses to preceding electrical stimulation, recorded in hard copy over time. Reasoning backward from the movement of the atrial or ventricular walls, and undulations of the atrioventricular and/or semilunar valves, to the preceding electrical event permits indirect analysis of the electrophysiology of the underlying rhythm[3–6].

Obtaining diagnostic tracings may be time-consuming, since the m-mode sampling line must be correctly oriented. Ideally, the m-mode cursor should transect the atria and ventricles simultaneously, allowing visualization of rate and atrioventricular contraction. This alignment is not always easy to obtain, and is heavily dependent on fetal position. Fetal movement and fetal breathing may also complicate the process.

Pulsed Doppler flow analysis may also be useful for analyzing fetal cardiac rhythm[7–11]. This technique involves recording intravascular or intracardiac blood flow in hard copy against time. Pulsed Doppler evaluation relates the flow patterns within the cardiovascular system to the mechanical, and therefore electrical, events immediately preceding. Signals representing flow across the atrioventricular junction in the fetus differ significantly from those seen postnatally[7]. Because the fetal ventricular myocardium is less compliant than that of the neonate or older child, the fetal heart is more dependent upon active atrial contraction for adequate ventricular filling[12]. The Doppler flow waveform of transmitral or transtricuspid valve flow thus shows less flow in the early, passive, filling phase (E wave) than in the active (A wave) portion of diastolic filling.

When pulsed Doppler flow analysis is used for fetal cardiac rhythm assessment, the sample volume can be placed in the left ventricle, at the junction of the ventricular inflow tract and outflow tract to the aortic outflow. Here both ventricular filling and emptying can be seen with inflow and outflow on opposite sides of the baseline, as the flow directions are opposite to one another. DeVore and Horenstein recently described a similar strategy[13], placing the Doppler sample volume in a position overlapping pulmonary venous and arterial flow. Similarly, the sample volume can be positioned to overlap the ascending aorta and the superior vena cava, which are adjacent to each other. Visualization of an early 'A' wave during diastole may identify early electrical stimulation of the fetal atrium. While we find the m-mode echocardiogram to be more helpful and understandable than pulsed Doppler tracings for rhythm analysis, Doppler evaluation has provided information regarding the physiologic impact of fetal arrhythmias on the fetal cardiovascular system[10].

## THE IRREGULAR FETAL HEART RATE

The most common indication for fetal rhythm analysis is an irregular fetal heart rate. Variable fetal heart rate decelerations are common in the second trimester, especially while the patient lies supine[14], so it is important to distinguish transient slowing of the fetal heart from a true irregularity. The former is benign and does not require further investigation, while the latter, most often also benign, warrants further evaluation.

The most common irregularity of fetal cardiac rhythm occurs irregularly, with a pattern that suggests a pause or an extra beat. A supraventricular extrasystole occurring very early in diastole may occur during the atrioventricular conduction system's refractory period and is not conducted into the ventricle to initiate a ventricular response. The atrial pacemaker is reset, resulting in a longer pause between ventricular ejections than normal. The absence of ejection into the fetal arteries results in a skipped beat being heard, even though the underlying electrophysiology actually is that of an early extra beat. Doppler flow analysis demonstrates passive E wave filling of the ventricle after ventricular systole, with the early A wave appearing close to, or even superimposed upon, the E wave. If the premature A wave is not obscured in the passive filling phase, the time to the next A wave can be seen to be the same as between normal beats.

If a supraventricular extrasystole occurs slightly later in diastole it may enter the atrioventricular conduction system at a time when conduction into the ventricle can occur, but even then diastolic filling of the ventricle may be insufficient for significant ejection of blood into the fetal arteries. Auscultation may note a weak premature beat, or no pulse at all – again leading to the perception of a pause rather than an extra beat. Typically the post-extrasystolic beat is more forceful than usual[10], because of enhanced diastolic ventricular preload during the prolonged diastolic filling period. This increased diastolic volume enhances ventricular ejection in the intact fetal ventricle via the Frank–Starling mechanism[12,15]. The longer diastolic run-off period during the post-extrasystolic pause, leads to lower diastolic arterial pressures. Therefore the first post-extrasystolic beat occurs in a setting of enhanced fetal ventricular preload and decreased afterload. The fetus without a potentiated post-extrasystolic beat may be considered to have intrinsic impairment of ventricular myocardium (Figure 1).

Determining the level within the heart where isolated extrasystoles arise (i.e. atrial versus junctional versus ventricular), is time-consuming and often difficult, and occasionally impossible. These efforts appear to have little pragmatic significance, since the isolated extrasystole is of importance only as a potential clue to the risk of sustained tachyarrhythmias in the future[16]. In such cases the usual underlying mechanism involves re-entry circuits, either within areas of diseased atrial or ventricular myocardium, or, more frequently, involving accessory conduction pathways at the level of the atrioventricular junction[1]. We have noted the onset of sustained fetal or neonatal supraventricular tachycardia in only five fetuses out of almost 1200 fetuses who were determined to have isolated extrasystoles (approximately

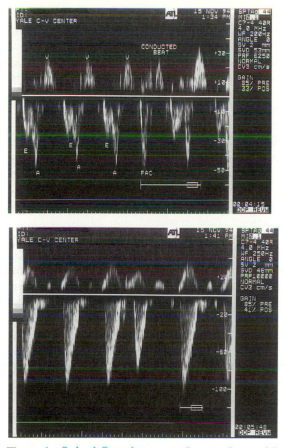

**Figure 1** Pulsed Doppler waves from a fetus with premature atrial beats. Top panel, sample volume placed in the fetal left ventricle. Waves below the baseline represent biphasic ventricular filling (E, A). Note early A wave in premature atrial contraction (PAC). Flow above the baseline is ejection into the aorta with ventricular systole (V). The PAC is conducted with a smaller flow-velocity wave than those seen after the normal beats. Bottom panel, sample volume placed in the aortic arch. Note that wave from conducted premature beat occurs early, and is smaller than the normal waves. Subsequent wave is larger, representing post-extrasystolic potentiation due to increased preload and diminished afterload

0.4%). Four of these occurred prenatally, the fifth occurred on the 3rd postnatal day in a neonate who was diagnosed as having blocked atrial bigeminy *in utero*, and had Wolff–Parkinson–White syndrome on the neonatal ECG. We have also evaluated a fetus who was originally referred for isolated extrasystoles and found to have brief runs of supraventricular tachycardia on fetal echocardiography.

Our recommendation for fetuses with extrasystoles is to have the fetal heart rate checked weekly until the irregularity resolves. The 1-week interval between checks minimizes the risk of developing non-immune hydrops from sustained fetal supraventricular tachycardia between visits. The fetus with frequent premature beats, or even atrial bigeminy, can be managed similarly.

We also recommend that the mother avoid sympathomimetic agents such as caffeine or β-adrenergic tocolytics. If preterm labor develops, alternative agents such as intravenous magnesium or oral nifedipine may be preferable.

The major complication of frequent extrasystoles is that they may make it difficult to monitor the fetal heart rate in labor. This can be circumvented with patience, and consideration of the long-term fetal heart rate pattern. We continue to recommend full fetal echocardiographic evaluation for all fetuses presenting with irregular fetal heart rates based on the small possibility that structural or functional abnormalities could underlie the extrasystoles. We have also seen fetuses with atrial flutter and variable block, and with brief episodes of re-entrant tachycardia who sound similar to the fetus with extrasystoles on external auscultation. Complications occurring to the fetus with isolated extrasystoles are rare, and isolated extrasystoles in the neonate or child tend to follow a benign course, which argue strongly against any attempt to suppress extrasystoles with maternal medications[17].

## SUPRAVENTRICULAR TACHYCARDIA

With the exception of sinus tachycardias, the most common fetal tachycardia is supraventricular tachycardia. This is most often of a reciprocating or atrioventricular re-entrant etiology. In this situation a circular movement of electrical impulses is initiated by an extrasystole which is conducted slowly through the atrioventricular node to the ventricle, then re-enters the atrial tissue through an accessory conduction pathway outside the atrioventricular node[1].

Reciprocating atrioventricular re-entrant tachycardia depends on the presence of an accessory pathway with a different conduction velocity and effective refractory period from the atrioventricular node. Antiarrhythmic therapy therefore involves a strategy of altering the conduction velocities and/or refractory periods of the atrioventricular nodal tissue (most frequently) and/or the accessory conduction tissue[1]. The rate of fetal atrioventricular reciprocating tachycardia is almost always 240–260 beats/min. Our experience suggests that any sustained tachycardia outside of this range is likely to represent an arrhythmia other than atrioventricular reciprocating tachycardia. On the other hand, the inverse statement, that any tachycardia in the 240–260 beats/min range must be atrioventricular reciprocating tachycardia cannot be made.

Determining the need for antiarrhythmic therapy must be based on a logical analysis of a number of factors, including gestational age, the presence or absence of fetal hydrops, and the relative amount of time spent in the tachycardia. A non-hydropic fetus with occasional non-sustained episodes of tachycardia at term should be delivered for postnatal evaluation and treatment. An hydropic mid-trimester fetus with an incessant tachycardia merits a completely different approach. Most patients, however, do not fall into either of these extremes, and the approach that is made must be individualized according to local experience with postnatal management of premature neonates with sustained cardiac arrhythmias. The dismal prognosis expected for severely hydropic premature infants suggests that many of these fetuses will be better candidates for *in utero* rather than postnatal therapy.

In the absence of fetal hydrops it has become our practice to monitor the fetus for a prolonged period, to establish the pattern of time spent in the tachycardia. This helps us determine whether fetal therapy is indicated, and whether initial doses of medication are having any effect on the frequency and duration of the arrhythmia.

Whether or not a fetus with intermittent tachycardia will develop hydrops is an important determinant of the need for fetal therapy. It is unclear why some fetuses take a prolonged period to develop hydrops while others seem to develop severe hydrops relatively rapidly. Critical factors include venous hydrostatic pressure and serum oncotic pressure. Doppler studies of inferior vena caval flow during atrial ectopy and during sustained supraventricular tachycardia demonstrate prominent retrograde flow into the hepatic circulation. We have also noted that fetuses who remain hydropic after conversion to sinus rhythm have marked hypoalbuminemia and hypo-osmolality. The low serum oncotic pressure may explain why agents such as furosemide do not appear to have a significant therapeutic role. Fetal hypoalbuminemia may be related to passive hepatic congestion and secondary impairment of hepatic synthetic function.

Another possible important factor is the site of initial atrial depolarization (e.g. left versus right atrium), which could alter atrial emptying. Initial depolarization of the left atrium would result in a transient increase in left atrial pressure above right, which could partially close the foramen ovale, trapping a larger amount of blood in the right heart[18]. This would, in turn, lead to significantly higher systemic venous pressure and make the fetus more prone to the development of hydrops. We have seen this in two fetuses, suggesting that this mechanism occurs in the human, just as atrial pacing studies in sheep fetuses have demonstrated that altering the location of atrial pacing (right versus left) alters ventricular outputs and flow distribution in dramatic fashion[19].

Reciprocating atrioventricular tachycardia can be treated postnatally with rapid-acting pharmacologic agents, such as adenosine, which cause transient atrioventricular block breaking the re-entry circuit, and an immediate break in the tachycardia[20], or esophageal or intracardiac overdrive pacing and/or electrical cardioversion. The latter treatments have no role in fetal therapy. External compression of the umbilical cord has been reported to cause transient breaks in fetal tachycardia[21,22], although it has been unsuccessful in our experience. Such maneuvers may be useful as diagnostic tests to determine whether the underlying electrophysiologic mechanism of the tachycardia is atrioventricular re-entrant, but we would not expect more than a transient reversion to sinus rhythm. Extrasystoles, which are almost always present, quickly cause the tachycardia to recur.

Typical pharmacologic agents for the treatment of re-entrant tachycardia depress conduction and prolong the effective refractory period of the atrioventricular node, and include cardiac glycosides (digoxin), β-blockers (propranolol), calcium-channel blockers (verapamil, diltiazem), and adenosine[1,23]. Type IA antiarrhythmic agents (quinidine, procainamide, disopyramide)[24] and IC agents (flecainide)[25-28] have their primary impact on the accessory conduction pathways. Amiodarone (a type III agent) has been reported to be useful in some fetuses, after maternal oral therapy or direct fetal intravenous administration[29,30]. The extremely protracted half-life and the potential danger of associated side-effects, including interference with normal fetal thyroid function[31,32], and on myocardial development[33], have led us to consider this as a medication of last resort.

It is not surprising that there are varying opinions regarding the best approach to fetal antiarrhythmic therapy. We disagree with seeking a single agent that will reliably treat all arrhythmias, an unrealistic goal considering the variability of response of accurately diagnosed arrhythmias postnatally. The complex interactions between drug disposition in the mother, the fetus and the placenta make it likely that most drugs will vary in bioavailability from patient to patient. Even the most widely used agent, digoxin, is known to have variable penetration to the fetus, particularly in the presence of non-immune hydrops[34-36].

Agents such as amiodarone and flecainide, which have generally been reserved for the treatment of life-threatening arrhythmias postnatally, for treatment of fetal arrhythmias has been justified based on the potential for fetal demise. Maternal administration of these agents causes significant blood levels in the mother, who is not herself in danger until she is exposed

to the potentially life-threatening proarrhythmic risks of these drugs[37]. The loss of a fetal patient is a tragedy for the parents and for the treating physician, but this would be dwarfed by an iatrogenic maternal death. For this reason agents with significant proarrhythmic potential (type IA, IC or III) should be used only in the presence of dire risk to the fetus, and only after informed consent is obtained from the parents. It is also essential that a team approach be employed, with appropriate counselling concerning both the mother and her fetus.

Our conclusion that digoxin was a logical drug to offer mothers for therapy of fetal supraventricular tachycardia was based on several considerations:

(1) It has been used for over two centuries;

(2) Its safety in pregnancy has been well documented over that time;

(3) It is widely available and inexpensive;

(4) It is a positive, rather than a negative, inotropic agent; and

(5) Assays for serum level are easily obtained.

Empirical use of this agent demonstrated its utility for use in postnatal supraventricular tachycardia and it proved to be quite effective in the therapy of fetal supraventricular tachycardia. Although digoxin does not control all supraventricular tachycardias, it remains our first line drug for fetal supraventricular tachycardia. In about 40% of cases a second agent is still required.

Verapamil was introduced as an important alternative for the treatment of neonatal re-entrant supraventricular tachycardia. This agent was quite effective and we used it as the second-line drug in our emerging algorithm. In 1987 Garson reported the potential for hemodynamic collapse in 10–20% of neonates receiving verapamil for the treatment of supraventricular tachycardia with congestive heart failure by intravenous push[38]. While we were not administering the agent intravenously to the mother, we certainly were administering it to immature patients with an immature, presumably calcium-flux-dependent, myocardium, and this led us to discontinue the use of verapamil. The speed at which agents such as verapamil change from magic bullets to evidence of malpractice is alarming, but highlights the need to remain abreast of changes in therapy, further emphasizing the importance of a multidisciplinary approach to such patients.

Flecainide, a type IC agent, was introduced as a potential remedy for all forms of supraventricular and ventricular tachycardia. A drug with a spectrum of antiarrhythmic activity so broad that the accuracy of the electrophysiologic diagnosis of the fetal arrhythmia becomes much less important is attractive. Flecainide has been useful for the treatment of a wide variety of pediatric and fetal arrhythmias[25–28]. Unfortunately, agents in this class were reported to cause proarrhythmic deaths when used as prophylaxis against ventricular arrhythmias after myocardial infarction[39], which led to an overall reconsideration of the use of type IC agents. Subsequent experience, especially in pediatrics[40], has suggested type IC drugs to be useful. The cardiovascular status of the older men surviving myocardial infarction who constituted the study population of the CAST study is quite different from the fetus and the mother, but the potential for a ventricular proarrhythmic effect of this agent definitely exists.

These experiences have even led to a re-examination of our most fundamental antiarrhythmic agent, digoxin. A 1% incidence of sudden death among children receiving digoxin for long-term treatment of supraventricular tachycardia in the presence of Wolff–Parkinson–White syndrome has been reported[41]. Those with the Wolff–Parkinson–White syndrome receiving digoxin are at risk of shortened antegrade effective refractory period in the accessory pathway, which may cause a fatal rapid conduction of intercurrent atrial fibrillation[42]. Some have suggested that digoxin not be used at all in the face of Wolff–Parkinson–White syndrome at any age[43]. Gillette and colleagues have suggested that if the effective refractory period is above 220 ms during treatment, infants may be safely treated with digoxin, even in the presence of Wolff–Parkinson–White syndrome. They point out that this agent has been used for

years for neonatal supraventricular tachycardia and that empirical experience shows that it works[44]. We still consider digoxin our drug of first choice when reciprocating atrioventricular tachycardia requires treatment in the fetus, although we are not able to exclude Wolff–Parkinson–White syndrome in these fetuses, and we certainly are unable to measure the length of the effective refractory period.

Pregnant women can be demonstrated to have digoxin-like immunoreactive substance (DLIS) in their serum, especially in the presence of polyhydramnios and hydrops fetalis, and that DLIS is also present in the fetal circulation[34,45]. DLIS has been identified to be ouabain, with $Na^+$–$K^+$ ATP-ase blocking activity[46,47]. It has been suggested that maternally administered digoxin does not reach the hydropic fetus across an edematous placenta, in which case serum assays suggesting otherwise are confounded by DLIS[34–36]. It is unproven that maternal and/or fetal digoxin toxicity can be induced more easily when an exogenous drug is added to a system that is already producing endogenous ouabain. We are unaware of any cases in which such toxicity has been suggested.

The risks of treatment touched on above emphasize the importance of collaboration between obstetric and pediatric cardiology consultants in the treatment of fetal arrhythmias. Indications for therapy and drug selection should be based on an understanding of the electrophysiology of the arrhythmia and the pharmacology and pharmacokinetics of the agents being employed. Sequential administration of drugs should be based on an understanding of the mechanism of drug action. Using agents that act through similar mechanisms only increases the potential for disastrous proarrhythmic side-effects with no added benefit. A published algorithm has suggested that the secondline of therapy of hydropic fetuses with sustained supraventricular tachycardia who are unresponsive to digoxin should be the simultaneous maternal administration of procainamide and quinidine[48]. Both of these type IA drugs may cause proarrhythmic effects leading to fatal Torsades de Pointes secondary to pathologic prolongation of the QT interval. The use of these agents in combination is rare and controversial, and a mix that most electrophysiologists would consider potentially lethal to both mother and fetus.

Supraventricular tachycardia with hydrops is usually treated as an emergency with the expectation that the tachycardia should be controlled as rapidly as possible. Although some fetuses may die soon after diagnosis, and we have had one patient have a fetal demise within an hour of arrival, before therapy could be instituted, in general these fetuses are not moribund, and may be safely observed and treated in a logical fashion. Antiarrhythmic agents may require hours or days to reach therapeutic levels in the fetus. Equally important, many of these agents (e.g. flecainide and amiodarone) have long half-lives, remaining in the mother or fetus long after treatment might be discontinued. There should be a logical sequence followed if medications are to be changed, in order to avoid the potential toxicity of having multiple antiarrhythmic agents in the body at the same time.

We currently use digoxin as our first-line agent to treat reciprocating supraventricular tachycardia in the preterm hydropic fetus. We use an intravenous loading dose of 1.0 mg divided over 12 hours (0.5/0.25/0.25 mg at 6-hour intervals) after obtaining maternal electrolytes and an electrocardiogram, and have the mother on continuous cardiac monitoring. The fetus is observed by continuous external electronic monitoring and fetal ultrasound is performed at least daily.

We initiate all fetal antiarrhythmic therapy on an inpatient basis. Incremental intravenous doses of digoxin are frequently required, and the total loading dose over the first 24–36 hours of treatment may be as high as 2.0 mg. Oral maintenance therapy is then instituted, again monitoring for electrocardiographic or subjective evidence of maternal digoxin toxicity. We seek to reach maternal serum digoxin levels at the upper end of the therapeutic range, which often requires surprisingly high digoxin doses (0.50–1.0 mg/day). If other medications are ultimately needed, it is essential to remember that some antiarrhythmic agents (quinidine, verapamil and amiodarone) increase digoxin

serum levels and bioavailability, even if digoxin doses and levels have previously been stable. Before initiating these other drugs, the mother's digoxin dose should be empirically cut by 50% or more, to prevent digoxin toxicity.

Lack of response may be due to inadequate delivery of drug to the (fetal) patient or because the arrhythmia has been incorrectly diagnosed. The differential diagnosis of fetal atrial tachycardia includes ectopic focus tachycardia, in which the heart rate arises from an irritable focus of atrial tissue. This inappropriate and rapid pacemaker usurps the normal sinus pacemaker, and results in an incessant tachycardia[49]. Approximately 10% of fetal and neonatal tachycardia are due to this mechanism, which is extremely difficult to treat and may not respond to any standard medical approaches. Digoxin may induce atrioventricular block, but that alone does not break these tachycardias. Adenosine, verapamil, pacing and electrical cardioversion are also ineffective, although the type IA, IC II (β-blockers), or III classes of drugs may be useful for ectopic focus tachycardia.

## ATRIAL FLUTTER/FIBRILLATION

Atrial flutter and fibrillation are less common in the fetus than supraventricular tachycardia (Table 1), similarly to their relative frequencies in newborns. Non-immune hydrops is common, and there is a high mortality rate (Table 2) reflecting both difficulty in controlling these

**Table 1** Fetal cardiac arrhythmias – Yale experience

| | |
|---|---|
| Isolated extrasystoles | 1026 |
| Supraventricular tachycardia | 58 |
| Atrial flutter | 17 |
| Atrial fibrillation | 2 |
| Sinus tachycardia | 6 |
| Junctional tachycardia | 1 |
| Ventricular tachycardia | 7 |
| Complete heart block | 29 |
| Second-degree atrioventricular block | 8 |
| Sinus bradycardia | 6 |
| Total | 1160 |

**Table 2** Fetal tachycardias – outcomes

| | |
|---|---|
| Supraventricular (re-entrant) tachycardia ($n = 58$) | |
| gestational age | 19–39 weeks |
| hydrops fetalis | 32 |
| congenital heart disease | 1 |
| deaths | 3 |
| Atrial flutter ($n = 17$) | |
| gestational age | 24–38 weeks |
| hydrops fetalis | 9 |
| congenital heart disease | 5 |
| deaths | 4 |
| Atrial fibrillation ($n = 2$) | |
| gestational age | 19–38 weeks |
| hydrops fetalis | 0 |
| congenital heart disease | 0 |
| deaths | 0 |

rhythms prenatally and a relatively greater frequency of structural heart disease.

Atrial flutter results from a circular re-entrant movement of electrical energy within the atrium, with rates usually in the range of 400–480 beats/min. Varying degrees of atrioventricular block are present, leading to varying ventricular response rates, which may be fixed and unresponsive to fetal activity (for example, if fixed 2 : 1 atrioventricular block is present) or highly irregular (if there is variable atrioventricular block). The presence of atrioventricular block is further evidence that atrioventricular re-entry via the atrioventricular node is not the underlying electrophysiologic mechanism of atrial flutter.

Postnatal therapy of atrial flutter is based on controlling the ventricular response rate, to decrease the degree of heart failure prior to conversion of the flutter to sinus rhythm. In situations in which sinus rhythm is not achieved, simple control of ventricular response rate may be the therapeutic goal. We have found prenatal control of ventricular response rate alone in hydropic fetuses with atrial flutter to be insufficient, probably due to fetal hemodynamics, with a restrictive ventricular myocardium and relatively volume-loaded right heart[12,15]. This suggests that the fetal cardiovascular decompensation which accompanies sustained supraventricular tachyarrhythmias reflects diastolic, rather than systolic, pump dysfunction.

Normal fetal ventricular function depends on an effective atrial pump. Failure to control atrial flutter results in elevated atrial pressures with dilatation of the failing atrial pump, leading to further increases in systemic venous pressure, and with additional retardation of the resolution of fetal hydrops. The goal of antiarrhythmic therapy for fetal atrial flutter must therefore be restoration of a normal 1 : 1 atrioventricular contraction sequence. This usually requires incorporation of a type I agent such as procainamide or flecainide after the ventricular response rate is controlled with digoxin. Careful attention to the maternal digoxin level is important. The corrected QT interval of the maternal ECG must also be monitored until a stable dosage regimen is established.

Fetal atrial fibrillation appears to be even less common than atrial flutter. Our two cases responded to digoxin therapy alone, but if the arrhythmia had persisted we would have added a type I antiarrhythmic agent, for the same reasons as for atrial flutter.

The high mortality rate in our series of atrial flutter/fibrillation (4/19 [21%]) reflects the presence of congenital heart disease (5/19 cases). In all of these cases (two with critical pulmonary outflow obstruction and tricuspid insufficiency, one with Ebstein malformation of the tricuspid valve with severe tricuspid insufficiency and one with left atrial isomerism, atrioventricular valve insufficiency and complete heart block) marked atrial dilatation was present. The four deaths in our series included three of the patients with structural heart disease. In comparison, only one patient in our 58 cases of fetal reciprocating supraventricular tachycardia had congenital cardiac disease, a prematurely closed foramen ovale.

## VENTRICULAR TACHYCARDIA

We have diagnosed ventricular tachycardia rarely in the fetus, with seven prospective diagnoses. In each case, the heart rate during the tachycardia did not fall into the usual 240–260 beats/min range seen with atrioventricular reciprocating supraventricular tachycardia. Whenever the rate of fetal tachycardia falls outside of this range an unusual tachycardia must be considered. Atrioventricular dissociation was present in each of the fetuses in our series, although it is possible for fetuses with ventricular tachycardia to have retrograde conduction with a resulting 1 : 1 atrioventricular relationship.

Neonates with ventricular tachycardia are not invariably ill, and treatment is often not required. Five of our fetal patients were not hydropic with structurally normal hearts, and were not treated *in utero*. None of these required neonatal antiarrhythmic therapy. Considering the infrequency of episodes of postnatal tachycardia, the lack of symptoms during tachycardia, and the rarity of associated structural heart disease, it has been our impression that conservative management of fetal ventricular tachycardia is appropriate.

A sixth fetal patient presented during labor with ventricular tachycardia associated with marked right atrial and ventricular dilatation. Therapy was deferred until after delivery. The right ventricular dilatation persisted after delivery, with congestive heart failure and prolonged episodes of ventricular tachycardia. Arrhythmogenic right ventricular dysplasia was diagnosed and successfully treated with intravenous lidocaine, followed by oral mexiletine.

Our final diagnosis of ventricular tachycardia occurred in a laboring patient who received intravenous ephedrine for maternal hypotension after receiving an epidural. The episode lasted less than 1 hour and spontaneously resolved prior to delivery without sequelae.

The diagnosis of ventricular tachycardia in a previable fetus with evidence of congestive cardiac failure, should prompt consideration of antiarrhythmic therapy. It is important to avoid digoxin. Strategies such as direct umbilical venous administration of lidocaine or procainamide, followed by maternal therapy with oral procainamide, flecainide, or propranolol should be considered. The combination of fetal umbilical treatment and maternal oral treatment with these potent drugs once again should underscore the critical need for a collaborative approach between obstetricians and cardiolo-

gists in managing these patients. It is also important to bear in mind that fetuses with arrhythmias thought to be atrioventricular re-entry tachycardia with atypical rates may, in fact, be in ventricular tachycardia with 1 : 1 retrograde atrial activation, in which case digoxin would be contraindicated. Distinguishing these two possibilities may be difficult, if not impossible, in the absence of an ECG, although absence of the characteristic premature atrial beats triggering the runs of tachycardia or unusual rates of the tachycardia should raise concern about this possibility.

## SINUS TACHYCARDIA

Mild fetal tachycardia (180–210 beats/min) is usually not due to a primary cardiac electrophysiologic abnormality. The usual possible causes should be considered for fetuses with apparent sinus tachycardia, always remembering that ventricular tachycardia with 1 : 1 retrograde conduction may also present in this way. Maternal fever or bacterial intrauterine infection are important causes of sinus tachycardia, as is fetal distress, which can cause tachycardia with loss of beat-to-beat variability. Maternal or fetal hyperthyroidism can also cause fetal tachycardia. If that is a possibility, fetal goiter can be excluded with ultrasound. Finally, medications known to cause fetal tachycardia, such as β-mimetics (ritodrine, terbutaline), should be excluded. In each of these examples, it is more important to treat the underlying cause than to treat the tachycardia *per se*.

## BRADYCARDIAS

Significant fetal bradycardia can be defined as a fetal heart rate persistently below 100 beats/min. Sinus bradycardia is uncommon in the fetus; we have seen only six cases, none with rates lower than 90 beats/min. To establish this diagnosis, 1 : 1 atrioventricular concordance must be present, and some heart rate variability should be present. Intermittent fetal heart rate slowing should be evaluated by traditional obstetric criteria for the presence of significant decelerations requiring prompt intervention, rather than waiting for a fetal echocardiogram. A quick general ultrasound examination of the patient with persistent fetal bradycardia demonstrating good fetal movement and obvious atrioventricular discordance can avert an emergency Cesarean delivery and then be followed by appropriate cardiac evaluation. The patient having apparent episodic fetal bradycardia along with an irregular fetal heart rate usually is found to have atrial premature beats with periods of fetal atrial bigeminy during which every other beat is premature and is blocked at the atrioventricular node. This can be distinguished from Mobitz type II second-degree atrioventricular block or from complete heart block by observing the irregularity of the premature atrial contractions, in contrast to the regular atrial rate found with Mobitz type II second-degree block or complete heart block.

## COMPLETE HEART BLOCK

Approximately half of fetuses with complete heart block have underlying complex structural cardiac anomalies involving the atrioventricular junction. Visceral heterotaxy with left atrial isomerism and atrioventricular discordance are the most common findings. Complete heart block in association with severe structural heart disease is usually poorly tolerated by the fetus, especially when atrioventricular valve regurgitation is present; this combination is frequently associated with non-immune hydrops. It is rare for a fetus with hydrops, structural heart disease and complete heart block to survive[50–53].

Fetuses with complete heart block and structurally normal hearts are affected by an immunologically mediated process initiated by maternal autoantibodies[54–59]. These antibodies, initially described in Sjögren syndrome, are called anti-SSA and anti-SSB, also known respectively as anti-Ro and anti-La. They have a particularly strong affinity for the fetal cardiac conduction system, provoking an intense immune response. The antibodies also bind to fetal cardiac myocytes, and an immune myocarditis can also be demonstrated[60]. The frequent development of non-immune hydrops in fetuses with this form of heart block may be the result of a number of causes. The combination of a sudden drop in fetal ventricular rate and lack of co-ordination between the fetal atria and ventricles is poorly tolerated because the fetal heart is heavily reliant on active atrial contraction for normal ventricular filling. Fetal myocarditis further reduces ventricular compliance, thus increasing the reliance of the heart on co-ordinated atrial contraction for adequate ventricular filling.

Several treatment approaches have been reported for fetal heart block. A surgical approach has been suggested for placement of a fetal pacemaker. The feasibility of percutaneous pacemaker lead placement and transient ventricular capture has been reported, although the fetus was moribund when the procedure was undertaken and there was little fetal response[61]. A report of transvenous ventricular pacing has also appeared, with only transient ventricular pacing without fetal survival[62]. An attempt by a group at the University of California, San Francisco, in an open procedure, was similarly unsuccessful (Harrison M., personal communication). For direct fetal pacing to succeed, better fetal surgical techniques will be needed. Ventricular pacing alone may be insufficient, because it may be necessary to achieve sequential atrioventricular pacing to eliminate the 'cannon a waves' that elevate fetal atrial and venous pressures and impede resorption of fetal edema. The pacemaker itself would need to be placed in such a way as to avoid having free-floating wires in the amniotic fluid. Freely floating wires could be hazardous to the fetus if the umbilical cord became intertwined with them, similarly to the umbilical cord entanglement seen in monoamniotic twins. The ideal surgical solution would be a sequential atrioventricular pacemaker placed subcutaneously in the fetus or threaded through the umbilical cord from the placental insertion, either of which represents a formidable technical challenge.

Fetuses with second-degree heart block may progress to have complete heart block, suggesting a possible medical treatment for these fetuses. Plasmapheresis and corticosteriods have been among the treatments suggested in the past[63–65], although the steroid used most often in the past was prednisone, which crosses the placenta poorly. We reasoned that selecting a steroid that crosses the placenta efficiently, and treating early in the course of the disease might ameliorate the myocarditis, and might even improve the rhythm. We also noted that the onset of immune fetal heart block was usually at about 20–24 weeks' gestation, and has not been reported earlier than 17–18 weeks' gestation. This coincides with the development of responsiveness of the fetal immune system. This is analogous to fetal syphilis and viral infections, which may cross the placenta without provoking a fetal response until some immune competence develops, further suggesting that immune suppression might be a useful approach.

We have treated five fetuses with maternal dexamethasone (4 mg *per os* four times a day) and have seen evidence of fetal responses in four[66]. Two fetuses completely resolved non-immune hydrops, and one of these transiently reverted to second-degree atrioventricular block. One additional fetus, presenting with second-degree block and high maternal anti-SSA/Ro and anti-SSB/La titers, reverted to first-degree block. One fetus presenting in mixed second- and third-degree block is stable postnatally in second-degree block. These results are encouraging, although the resolution of fetal hydrops may just have coincided with the treatment, as the fetal myocardium adjusted to the atrio-ventricular dissociation. We have never observed immune-mediated fetal heart block to improve spontaneously, nor has it been reported in the literature, suggesting that the effects are real. A randomized multicenter trial will be necessary to confirm the benefits of this treatment.

## CONCLUSIONS

We have reviewed the common fetal arrhythmias, their pathogenesis and treatments. Prior to any intrauterine therapy the underlying principles we have outlined should be considered:

(1) The underlying accurate diagnosis of the abnormality;

(2) The need for intrauterine therapy compared to delivery;

(3) The risks and benefits of therapy;

(4) Appropriate maternal and fetal monitoring of therapy; and

(5) Obtaining fully informed consent.

These decisions require extensive discussions with patients, and cannot be undertaken unilaterally by physicians, and furthermore, require close collaboration between cardiologists and obstetricians for optimal results. We believe that such efforts are best reserved for tertiary centers, as for invasive fetal therapies, to concentrate the experience and skills that are needed to provide the best outcomes. The institution providing care should also be prepared to care for any maternal or fetal complications that may ensue. The field of fetal arrhythmia therapy has been one of the earliest examples of fetal treatment, and its successes can be a model for other areas of fetal therapy, if we bear these principles in mind.

# References

1. Kleinman, C. S. and Copel, J. A. (1991). Electrophysiologic principles and fetal antiarrhythmic therapy. *Ultrasound Obstet. Gynecol.*, **1**, 286–97

2. Kleinman, C. S. and Copel, J. A. (1996). Diagnosis and treatment of fetal supraventricular tachycardia. *Prog. Pediatr. Cardiol.*, in press

3. Kleinman, C. S., Hobbins, J. C., Jaffe, C. C. *et al.* (1980). Echocardiographic studies of the human fetus: prenatal diagnosis of congenital heart disease and cardiac dysrhythmias. *Pediatrics*, **65**, 1059–67

4. Kleinman, C. S., Donnerstein, R. L., Jaffe, C. C. *et al.* (1983). Fetal echocardiography, a tool for evaluation of *in utero* cardiac arrhythmias and monitoring of *in utero* therapy: analysis of 71 patients. *Am. J. Cardiol.*, **51**, 237–43

5. DeVore, G. R., Siassi, B. and Platt, L. D. (1983). Fetal echocardiography III. The diagnosis of car-

diac arrhythmias using real-time-directed M-mode ultrasound. *Am. J. Obstet. Gynecol.*, **146**, 792–9

6. Silverman, N. H., Enderlein, M. A., Stanger, P. *et al.* (1985). Recognition of fetal arrhythmias by echocardiography. *J. Clin. Ultrasound*, **13**, 255–63

7. Kleinman, C. S., Weinstein, E. M. and Copel, J. A. (1986). Pulsed Doppler analysis of human fetal blood flow. *Clin. Diagn. Ultrasound*, **17**, 173–85

8. Strasburger, J. F., Huhta, J. C., Carpenter, R. J. *et al.* (1986). Doppler echocardiography in the diagnosis and management of persistent fetal arrhythmias. *J. Am. Coll. Cardiol.*, **7**, 1386–91

9. Steinfeld, L., Rappaport, H. L., Rossbach, H. C. and Martinez, E. (1986). Diagnosis of fetal arrhythmias using echocardiographic and Doppler techniques. *J. Am. Coll. Cardiol.*, **7**, 1425–33

10. Reed, K. L., Sahn, D. J., Marx, G. R. *et al.* (1987). Cardiac Doppler flows during fetal arrhythmias: physiologic consequences. *Obstet. Gynecol.*, **70**, 1–6

11. Lingman, G. and Marsál, K. (1987). Fetal cardiac arrhythmias: Doppler assessment. *Semin. Perinatol.*, **11**, 357–61

12. Romero, T., Covell, J. W. and Friedman, W. F. (1972). A comparison of pressure–volume relations of the fetal, newborn and adult heart. *Am. J. Physiol.*, **222**, 1285–90

13. DeVore, G. R. and Horenstein, J. (1993). Simultaneous Doppler recording of the pulmonary artery and vein: a new technique for the evaluation of a fetal arrhythmia. *J. Ultrasound Med.*, **12**, 669–71

14. Sorokin, Y., Bottoms, S. F., Dierker, L. J. and Rosen, M. G. (1982). The clustering of fetal heart rate changes and fetal movements in pregnancies between 20 and 30 weeks of gestation. *Am. J. Obstet. Gynecol.*, **143**, 952–7

15. Rudolph, A. M. (1974). *Congenital Diseases of the Heart.* (Chicago: Yearbook)

16. Kleinman, C. S. and Copel, J. A. (1994). Fetal cardiac arrhythmias: diagnosis and therapy. In Creasy, R. K. and Resnick, R. (eds.) *Maternal–Fetal Medicine, Principles and Practice*, 3rd edn., pp. 326–41. (Philadelphia: W. B. Saunders)

17. Blandon, R. and Leandro, I. (1984). Fetal heart arrhythmia: clinical experience with antiarrhythmic drugs. In Doyle, E. F., Engle, M. A., Gersony, W. M., Rashkind, W. J. and Talner, N. S. (eds.) *Pediatric Cardiology, Proceedings of the Second World Congress*, pp. 483–4. (New York: Springer-Verlag)

18. Buis-Liem, T. N., Ottenkamp, J., Meerman, R. H. and Verwey, R. (1987). The occurrence of fetal supraventricular tachycardia and obstruction of the foramen ovale. *Prenatal Diagn.*, **7**, 425–31

19. Nimrod, C., Davies, D., Harder, J. *et al.* (1987). Ultrasound evaluation of tachycardia-induced hydrops in the fetal lamb. *Am. J. Obstet. Gynecol.*, **157**, 655–9

20. Camm, A. J. and Garratt, C. J. (1991). Adenosine and supraventricular tachycardia. *N. Engl. J. Med.*, **325**, 1621–9

21. Martin, C. B., Nijhuis, J. G. and Weijer, A. A. (1984). Correction of fetal supraventricular tachycardia by compression of the umbilical cord. Report of a case. *Am. J. Obstet. Gynecol.*, **150**, 324–6

22. Fernandez, C., De Rosa, G. E., Guevara, E. *et al.* (1988). Reversion by vagal reflex of a fetal paroxysmal atrial tachycardia detected by echocardiography. *Am. J. Obstet. Gynecol.*, **159**, 860–1

23. Kleinman, C. S., Copel, J. A., Weinstein, E. M. *et al.* (1985). Treatment of fetal tachyarrhythmias. *J. Clin. Ultrasound*, **13**, 265–73

24. Gunteroth, W. G., Cyr, D. R., Mack, L. A. *et al.* (1985). Hydrops from reciprocating atrioventricular tachycardia in a 27-week fetus requiring quinidine for conversion. *Obstet. Gynecol.*, **66**, 29S–33S

25. Wren, C. and Hunter, S. (1988). Maternal administration of flecainide to terminate and suppress fetal tachycardia. *Br. Med. J.*, **296**, 249

26. Allan, L. D., Chita, S. K., Sharland, G. K. *et al.* (1991). Flecainide in the treatment of fetal tachycardias. *Br. Heart J.*, **65**, 46–8

27. Kofinas, A. D., Simon, N. V., Sagel, H. *et al.* (1991). Treatment of fetal supraventricular tachycardia with flecainide acetate after digoxin failure. *Am. J. Obstet. Gynecol.*, **165**, 630–1

28. Perry, J. C., Ayres, N. A. and Carpenter, R. J. (1991). Fetal supraventricular tachycardia treated with flecainide acetate. *J. Pediatr.*, **118**, 303–5

29. Arnoux, P., Seyral, P., Llurens, M. *et al.* (1987). Amiodarone and digoxin for refractory fetal tachycardia. *Am. J. Cardiol.*, **59**, 166–7

30. Gembruch, U., Manz, M., Bald, R. *et al.* (1989). Repeated intravascular treatment with amiodarone in a fetus with refractory supraventricular tachycardia and hydrops fetalis. *Am. Heart J.*, **118**, 1335–8

31. Laurent, M., Betremieux, P., Biron, P. and Le-Helloco, A. (1987). Neonatal hypothyroidism after treatment by amiodarone during pregnancy. *Am. J. Cardiol.*, **60**, 942

32. Rovet, J., Ehrlich, R. and Sorbara, D. (1987). Intellectual outcome in children with fetal hypothyroidism. *J. Pediatr.*, **110**, 700–4

33. Nag, A. C., Lee, M. L. and Shepard, D. (1990). Effect of amiodarone on the expression of myosin isoforms and cellular growth of cardiac muscle cells in culture. *Circulation Res.*, **67**, 51–60

34. Weiner, C. P., Landas, S. and Persoon, T. J. (1987). Digoxin-like immunoreactive substance in fetuses with and without cardiac pathology. *Am. J. Obstet. Gynecol.*, **157**, 368–71

35. Younis, J. S. and Granat, M. (1987). Insufficient transplacental digoxin transfer in severe hydrops fetalis. *Am. J. Obstet. Gynecol.*, **157**, 1268–9

36. Weiner, C. P. and Thompson, M. I. B. (1988). Direct treatment of fetal supraventricular tachycardia after failed transplacental therapy. *Am. J. Obstet. Gynecol.*, **158**, 570–3

37. Morganroth, J. (1987). Risk factors for the development of proarrhythmic events. *Am. J. Cardiol.*, **59**, 32E–37E

38. Garson, A. Jr. (1987). Medicolegal problems in the management of cardiac arrhythmias in children. *Pediatrics*, **79**, 84–8

39. The Cardiac Arrhythmia Suppression Trial (CAST) Investigators (1989). Preliminary report: effect of encainide and flecainide on mortality in a randomized trial of arrhythmia suppression after myocardial infarction. *N. Engl. J. Med.*, **3**, 406–12

40. Fish, F. A., Gillette, P. C. and Benson, D. W. Jr. (1991). Proarrhythmia, cardiac arrest and death in young patients receiving encainide and flecainide. *J. Am. Coll. Cardiol.*, **18**, 356–65

41. Deal, B. J., Kane, J. F., Gillette, P. C. *et al.* (1985). Wolff–Parkinson–White syndrome with supraventricular tachycardia during infancy: management and follow-up. *J. Am. Coll. Cardiol.*, **5**, 130–5

42. Wellens, H. J. J. and Durrer, D. (1973). Effect of digitalis on atrioventricular conduction and circus movement tachycardia in patients with the Wolff–Parkinson–White syndrome. *Circulation*, **47**, 1229–33

43. Duvernoy, W. F. C. (1977). Sudden death in Wolff–Parkinson–White syndrome. *Am. J. Cardiol.*, **39**, 472–8

44. Gillette, P. C., Blair, H. L. and Crawford, F. A. (1990). Preexcitation syndromes. In Garson, A. Jr. (ed.) *Pediatric Arrhythmias: Electrophysiology & Pacing*, pp. 376–77. (Philadelphia: WB Saunders)

45. González, A. R., Phelps, S. J., Cochran, E. B. and Sibai, B. M. (1987). Digoxin-like immunoreactive substance in pregnancy. *Am. J. Obstet. Gynecol.*, **157**, 660–4

46. Ebara, H., Suzuki, S., Nagashima, K. and Kuroume, Y. (1988). Natriuretic activity of digoxin-like immunoreactive substance extracted from cord blood. *Life Sci.*, **42**, 303–9

47. Morris, J. F., Poston, L., Wolfe, C. D. and Hilton, P. J. (1988). A comparison of endogenous digoxin-like immunoreactivity and sodium transport inhibitory activity in umbilical and venous serum. *Clin. Sci.*, **75**, 577–9

48. DeVore, G. R., Siassi, B. and Platt, L. D. (1990). The fetus with cardiac arrhythmias. In Harrison, M. R., Golbus, M. S. and Filly, R. A. (eds.) *The Unborn Patient: Prenatal Diagnosis and Treatment*, 2nd edn., pp. 249–63. (Philadelphia: WB Saunders)

49. Knudson, J. M., Kleinman, C. S., Copel, J. A. and Rosenfeld, L. E. (1994). Ectopic atrial tachycardia *in utero*. *Obstet. Gynecol.*, **84**, 686–9

50. Kleinman, C. S., Copel, J. A. and Hobbins, J. C. (1987). Combined echocardiographic and Doppler assessment of fetal congenital atrioventricular block. *Br. J. Obstet. Gynaecol.*, **94**, 967–74

51. Machado, M. V. L., Tynan, M. J., Curry, P. V. L. and Allan, L. D. (1988). Fetal complete heart block. *Br. Heart J.*, **60**, 512–15

52. Wladimiroff, J. W., Stewart, J. W. and Tonge, H. M. (1988). Fetal bradyarrhythmia: diagnosis and outcome. *Prenatal Diagn.*, **8**, 53–7

53. Schmidt, K. G., Ulmer, H. E., Silverman, N. H. *et al.* (1991). Perinatal outcome of fetal complete atrioventricular block: a multicenter experience. *J. Am. Coll. Cardiol.*, **17**, 1360–6

54. Chamiedes, L., Truex, R. C., Vetter, V. *et al.* (1977). Association of maternal systemic lupus erythematosus with congenital complete heart block. *N. Engl. J. Med.*, **297**, 1204–7

55. Esscher, E. and Scott, J. S. (1979). Congenital heart block and maternal systemic lupus erythematosus. *Br. Med. J.*, **1**, 1235–8

56. Scott, J. S., Maddison, P. J., Taylor, P. V. *et al.* (1983). Connective tissue disease, antibodies to ribonucleoprotein, and congenital heart block. *N. Engl. J. Med.*, **309**, 209–12

57. Litsey, S. E., Noonan, J., O'Connor, W. N. *et al.* (1985). Maternal connective tissue disease and congenital heart block. Demonstration of immunoglobulin in cardiac tissue. *N. Engl. J. Med.*, **312**, 98–100

58. Taylor, P. V., Scott, J. S., Gerlis, L. M. *et al.* (1986). Maternal antibodies against fetal cardiac antigens in congenital complete heart block. *N. Engl. J. Med.*, **315**, 667–72

59. Lee, L. A., Coulter, S., Erner, S. and Chu, H. (1987). Cardiac immunoglobulin deposition in congenital heart block associated with maternal anti-Ro antibodies. *Am. J. Med.*, **83**, 793–6

60. Horsfall, A. C., Venables, P. J. W., Taylor, P. V. and Maini, R. N. (1991). Ro and La antigens and maternal autoantibody idiotype in the surface of myocardial fibres in congenital heart block. *J. Autoimmun.*, **4**, 165–76

61. Carpenter, R. J., Strasburger, J. F., Garson, A. Jr. *et al.* (1986). Fetal ventricular pacing for hydrops secondary to complete atrioventricular block. *J. Am. Coll. Cardiol.*, **8**, 1434–6

62. Walkinshaw, S. A., Welch, C. R., McCormack, J. and Walsh, K. (1994). *In utero* pacing for fetal congenital heart block. *Fetal Diagn. Ther.*, **9**, 183–5

63. Buyon, J. P., Swersky, S. H., Fox, H. E. *et al.* (1986). Intrauterine therapy for presumptive fetal myocarditis with acquired heart block due to systemic lupus erythematosus. *Arth. Rheum.*, **30**, 44–9

64. Bierman, F. Z., Baxi, L., Jaffe, I. and Driscoll, J. (1988). Fetal hydrops and congenital complete heart block: response to maternal steroid therapy. *J. Pediatr.*, **112**, 646–8

65. Watson, W. J. and Katz, V. L. (1991). Steroid therapy for hydrops associated with antibody-mediated congenital heart block. *Am. J. Obstet. Gynecol.*, **165**, 553–4

66. Copel, J. A., Buyon, J. P. and Kleinman, C. S. (1995). Successful *in utero* treatment of fetal heart block. *Am. J. Obstet. Gynecol.*, **173**, 1384–90

# Prevalence and outcome of congenital heart disease in infancy: a 10-year population-based experience

## 10

*J. I. Brenner*

## INTRODUCTION

The clinical practice of pediatric cardiology has benefited from and been fundamentally changed by the advances in imaging technology, particularly ultrasound. Indeed, the entire practice of fetal cardiology has evolved over the last 15 years as a direct result of improved instrumentation. As a result of these technical advances, we can visualize details of cardiac anatomy in 16–18-week fetuses using the transabdominal approach, decipher major cardiac morphologic issues in 12–14-week fetuses using the transvaginal approach and investigate umbilical artery flow patterns in the fetus of 6–8 weeks' gestation. Practitioners of fetal cardiology have been prolific in describing their ever-increasing clinical experience. The writings are, in many cases, reminiscent of the initial phases of descriptive pediatric cardiology in the 1950s and 1960s, where center-based experience defines prevalence and outcome, and small case series expand the realm of possibility.

In an attempt to limit the bias inherent in the experience of a single center caring for the neonate and infant with congenital heart disease, researchers from several disciplines have approached the issues of prevalence and outcome in a variety of ways. In the USA, several large regional studies have been completed in the past two decades. In the 1970s, the New England Regional Infant Cardiac Program (NERICP) under the guidance of Dr Donald Fyler, served as a model to determine prevalence and evaluate resource utilization and clinical outcome, as well as report clinical descriptors of the birth cohort of infants referred to regional centers for care[1]. In the 1980s, the Baltimore–Washington Infant Study (BWIS) was created under the leadership of Dr Charlotte Ferencz, in an effort to investigate the etiologic determinants of congenital heart disease, employing the epidemiologic power provided by including both a cohort of infants with congenital heart disease and a control population from a fixed geographic area[2]. In addition to including a random sampling of live-born infants, the BWIS was unique in that there was a search of hospital logs and medical examiners' records in an effort to capture every infant with congenital heart disease born in the region during a defined period. The efforts to establish full ascertainment and inclusion of those with the most severe and therefore life-threatening defects were vital to the description of the birth cohort.

This effort to be all-inclusive strengthens the BWIS data set but also underscores the difficulty in describing the population of fetuses with congenital heart disease. We must recognize that only the most severe spectrum of cardiac dysmorphology is visible in the fetal population. For this reason, utilizing a case set of live-born infants with congenital heart disease and the attendant non-cardiac malformations may provide our best opportunity to understand the potential scope of the problem. What is the prevalence of congenital heart disease in a fixed geographic region with 'full' ascertainment of live-born infants? As a corollary, has the advent of pre-natal diagnosis made an impact on live-born prevalence during the BWIS data acquisition period? What are the major associated anomalies seen in infants with congenital heart disease that may influence management and survival? Lastly, what becomes of these infants during their first year of life?

This report will attempt to answer these questions. The full report of the Baltimore Washington Infant Study, *Epidemiology of Congenital Heart Disease: the BWIS 1981–1989*, was published in 1993 and contains the work of many of the dozens of participants in this decade long co-operative effort[2]. The research design, data collection, statistical methods, risk factor analysis and findings related to fetal, paternal and maternal exposure are all available for review. The reader is referred to this text for more comprehensive information. In this manuscript, I will emphasize only the case infant description.

## PREVALENCE AND THE RELATIONSHIP TO A FETAL POPULATION

During the years 1981–1989, there were 906 626 infants born in the BWIS region. Of these, 4390 infants (0.48%) were confirmed by echocardiography, cardiac catheterization, cardiac surgery, or autopsy to have congenital heart disease and were enrolled in the BWIS. Only 76 of 4390 infants (1.7%) were identified by review of autopsy logs (i.e. community search). All other infants were diagnosed in one of six cardiac regional centers. In addition, 3572 control infants were enrolled from the birth cohort.

The distribution of cases is seen in Table 1. As in other studies, ventricular septal defect predominates, accounting for 32% of infants with congenital heart disease. When combined with pulmonary valve stenosis (9%) and secundum atrial septal defects (7.7%), nearly half of the infant population with congenital heart disease is described. Of note, is the fact that this is not the population readily defined prenatally.

**Table 1** Frequency of congenital heart disease in the BWIS 1981–1989

|  | n | % |
|---|---|---|
| Ventricular septal defect | 1411 | 32.1 |
| Pulmonary stenosis | 395 | 9.0 |
| Atrial septal defect, secundum | 340 | 7.7 |
| Atrioventricular septal defect | 326 | 7.4 |
| Tetralogy of Fallot | 297 | 6.8 |
| Complete transposition | 208 | 4.7 |
| Coarctation of aorta (Coarc) | 203 | 4.6 |
| Hypoplastic left heart syndrome | 167 | 3.8 |
| Aortic stenosis | 128 | 2.9 |
| Patent arterial duct | 104 | 2.4 |
| Heterotaxy | 99 | 2.3 |
| Double outlet right ventricle | 86 | 2.0 |
| Bicuspid aortic valve | 84 | 1.9 |
| Pulmonary atresia with intact septum | 73 | 1.7 |
| Total anomalous pulmonary venous return | 60 | 1.4 |
| Common arterial trunk | 51 | 1.2 |
| Corrected (*1*) transposition | 47 | 1.1 |
| Ebstein anomaly | 43 | 1.0 |
| Tricuspid atresia | 32 | 0.7 |
| Interrupted aortic arch | 31 | 0.7 |
| Double inlet ventricle | 18 | 0.4 |
| Divided left atrium (cor triatriatum) | 5 | 0.1 |
| Other miscellaneous problems | 182 | 4.2% |

**Table 2**  Recognition prior to 1 week of age

|  | Total n | < 1 week n (%) |
|---|---|---|
| Pulmonary atresia | 73 | 58 (79.5) |
| Transposition | 208 | 165 (79.3) |
| Ebstein's anomaly | 43 | 33 (76.7) |
| Hypoplastic left heart | 167 | 123 (73.7) |
| Tricuspid atresia | 32 | 21 (65.6) |
| Interrupted aortic arch | 31 | 18 (58.1) |
| Heterotaxy | 99 | 57 (57.6) |
| Double inlet ventricle | 18 | 10 (58.6) |
| Common arterial trunk | 51 | 28 (54.9) |
| Total | 722 | |

**Table 3**  Recognition after 12 weeks of age

|  | Total n | > 12 weeks n (%) |
|---|---|---|
| Atrial septal defect | 340 | 153 (45.0) |
| Patent ductus arteriosus | 104 | 42 (40.4) |
| Pulmonary valve stenosis | 395 | 158 (40.0) |
| Aortic valve stenosis | 212 | 62 (29.2) |
| Ventricular septal defect | | |
| membranous | 896 | 181 (20.2) |
| muscular | 429 | 64 (14.9) |
| Total | 2376 | |

The lesions most often recognized prior to 1 week of age closely resemble the case list from published fetal experience (Table 2). Abnormalities of ventricular inflow, unequal septation and outflow atresia are strongly represented. Only transposition of the great arteries with its profound hemodynamic impact despite a normal four-chamber appearance, is an exception.

On the other hand, the structural abnormalities likely to be identified later in infancy, after 12 weeks of age, would only occasionally be identified by current fetal diagnostic practice (Table 3). The presence of a normal four-chamber view, along with the variability in onset of flow disturbance in obstructive lesions and the limitations of color flow imaging in utero, make the recognition of pulmonary stenosis, aortic stenosis and ventricular septal defects problematic. Normal in utero flow dynamics make definition of future persistence of ductal patency and atrial septal defects of the secundum variety all

but impossible. This group comprises 54.1% (2376/4390) of the study population.

The prevalence of congenital heart disease in the region appeared to increase from 1981 through 1989. As can be seen in Figure 1, the rate increased from 38/10 000 live births initially to 54/10 000 live births by the last years of registration. As pointed out by Martin and colleagues[3], nearly all of the increase can be accounted for by improved detection of 'minor' malformations, particularly ventricular septal defects of the muscular type. Color flow technology became widely available in the study region from 1986, accounting for the dramatic rise in the detection of muscular ventricular septal defects, which eventually constituted 44% of all ventricular septal defects defined in the latter 3-year period of the study.

While inclusion criteria did not change during the period of patient registration, the change in technology did have a major impact. The early assumption that only the most severe cases of congenital heart disease were recognized earlier became less valid as the study progressed. Eighty per cent of all cases were enrolled by 12 weeks of age, largely because of the ability of Doppler and color flow technology to define flow disturbance in the face of minimal morphologic abnormality.

Another factor impacting on the natural prevalence of congenital heart disease at live birth, alluded to in the introduction, was the impact of clinical fetal cardiology developing in the region during the latter years of infant registration in the BWIS. Comparison of the prevalence of two lethal malformations, transposition of the great arteries and hypoplastic left heart syndrome, reinforces the realization that prenatal detection impacts on postnatal experience. The absolute number of cases and the prevalence of transposition of the great arteries, with and without associated non-cardiac malformations remained fairly constant over the period 1981–1989, whereas the number of cases of hypoplastic left heart syndrome decreased 28% during the same period (Figure 2). The relative ease of prenatal detection of hypoplastic left heart syndrome compared to transposition of

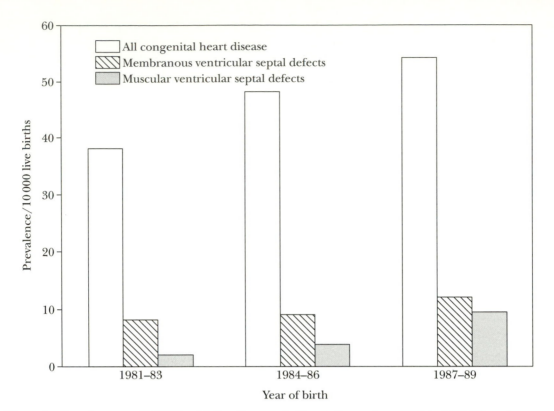

**Figure 1** Prevalence per 10 000 live births of congenital heart disease from 1981 to 1989. There is an overall increase from 38 to 54/10 000 but note cases with ventricular septal defects of the muscular type (2/10 000 in 1981–83 to 9.5/10 000 in 1987–89)

the great arteries, combined with current parental counseling and the selection of elective termination of pregnancy, clearly have an impact on postnatal prevalence.

The improved and more widely applied technology utilized in the neonatal and infant population may explain, in part, the 44% increase in recognition of infants with tetralogy of Fallot of less than 1 year of age during the study. The more aggressive approach to diagnosis and therapy of infants with trisomy 21 no doubt accounts for the trend towards earlier diagnosis, particularly of infants with partial forms of atrioventricular septal defects, atrial septal defects and other non-life-threatening malformations. Indeed, the reported prevalence of infants with Down syndrome and coexisting heart disease in this study is substantially higher than that recognized in the NERICP. Nearly 11% of the BWIS study population was made up of infants with

trisomy 21 whereas just over 5% of the population of the NERICP carried this diagnosis. This change reflects the evolution in ethical and cultural mores on medical practice in the USA as there almost certainly was not a doubling of the birth rate for infants with Down syndrome.

## CONGENITAL HEART DISEASE AND NON-CARDIAC MALFORMATIONS IN INFANCY

For the practicing pediatric cardiologist and for the investigator interested in the etiology of cardiac dysmorphology, one element of the BWIS has had a powerful impact. The recognition that the population of infants with congenital heart disease (cases) differs from their peer group (controls) by more than the presence of heart disease has opened up new avenues of thought and research into common etiologies.

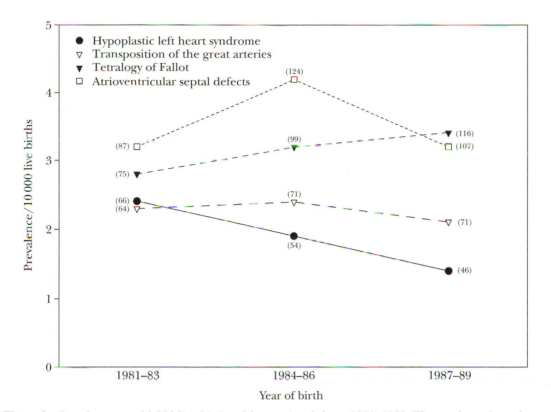

**Figure 2** Prevalence per 10 000 live births of four major defects, 1981–1989. The total number of cases in each time period is indicated in parentheses. Despite the increasing prevalence of congenital heart disease due to minor defects, tetralogy of Fallot in infancy was encountered more frequently from 1981 to 1983 than from 1987 to 1989, while hypoplastic left heart syndrome showed a substantial decline

Only 73% of infants with congenital heart disease had isolated heart malformations. In the control population, nearly 97% population had no abnormality. Non-cardiac malformations of all types were encountered eight times more frequently in cases. Most striking was the more than 100-fold increase in chromosomal abnormalities, using the conventional karyotyping techniques available in the 1980s. Chromosomal abnormalities constituted nearly one-half (522/1214) of all non-cardiac malformations. Interestingly, despite the trend to increased prenatal testing in obstetrical care established during the 1980s, the number of live-born infants with congenital heart disease and chromosomal abnormalities did not appear to decrease over time.

Table 4 highlights the non-cardiac malformations found in the BWIS case and control populations. Aneuploidy dominates the picture that developed in the 1980s. With the addition of fluorescent *in situ* hybridization technology, a shift from the 'syndromes' to the 'chromosomal' column in likely to occur in an important subset of infants. For example, the DiGeorge population (albeit only 30 cases recognized in 9 years), and probably other infants with cono-truncal abnormalities, will be discovered to have microdeletions explaining their multiple malformation sequences. This underscores the recognition of the critical role of single gene defects in the causation of congenital heart disease[4].

From the perspective of the fetal cardiologist, full ascertainment and therefore precise definition of the prevalence of congenital heart disease and chromosomal abnormality at 18 weeks remains an unobtainable goal. Clearly, prenatal recognition of atrioventricular septal defects,

111

**Table 4**  Case–control distribution of non-cardiac malformations

|  | Cases (n = 4390) | Controls (n = 3572) |
|---|---|---|
| I. No non-cardiac malformations | 3176 (72.3%) | 3452 (96.6%) |
| II. Chromosomal abnormalities | 522 (11.9%) | 3 (0.1%) |
| Down syndrome | 385 | 1 |
| III. Heritable syndromes | 327 (7.4%) | 21 (0.6%) |
| Ivemark | 68 |  |
| VACTERL | 37 |  |
| DiGeorge | 30 |  |
| IV. Non-heritable syndromes | 38 (0.86%) | 1 (0.03%) |
| V. Anomalies of organs | 229 (5.2%) | 36 (1.0%) |
| VI. Deformities, miscellaneous | 98 (2.2%) | 59 (1.7%) |

for example, is facilitated by the presence of coexisting clues on ultrasound: discrepancy in ventricular size (an unbalanced atrioventricular septal defect) producing an abnormal four-chamber view, or abnormality of outflow (double outlet right ventricle or tetralogy of Fallot), a more subtle finding during routine scanning. The uncommon but dramatic addition of complete heart block producing profound bradycardia would certainly prompt detailed fetal cardiac morphologic evaluation. Even the most common finding, trisomy 21 by amniocentesis, would be expected to produce a high yield of congenital heart disease during imaging study. However, despite these clues, prenatal ascertainment is far from complete. In the largest published series, Cook and co-workers[5] report 103 fetuses with atrioventricular septal defects, 17% of a population of 594 abnormal fetuses. Of these fetuses, only 34 (33%) had abnormal chromosomes. In contrast, the BWIS defined a live-born prevalence of atrioventricular septal defects of 7%, but 71% were found to have chromosomal abnormality, predominantly trisomy 21.

In an attempt to clarify the prenatal picture, Berg and colleagues[6] used accepted prenatal survival data to extrapolate back from a live-born population to fetal life. Assuming that 70% of fetuses with trisomy 21 will survive from 18 weeks to term, and recognizing 254 live-born infants with both trisomy 21 and atrioventricular septal defects in the BWIS population, an estimated 363 fetuses should be detectable by fetal ultrasound at 18 weeks' gestation

**Table 5**  High-risk lesions identifiable *in utero* based on live-born data from the BWIS

|  | % Abnormal |
|---|---|
| *Chromosomal abnormality* |  |
| Atrioventricular septal defect | 71 |
| Atrial septal defect | 14 |
| Coarctation of the aorta | 12 |
| Double outlet right ventricle | 12 |
| Tetralogy of Fallot | 11 |
| *Syndromes* |  |
| Heterotaxy | 65 |
| Interrupted aortic arch | 42 |
| Truncus arteriosus | 26 |
| *l*-Transposition of the great arteries | 23 |
| Double outlet right ventricle | 16 |
| *Organ malformations* |  |
| Tetralogy of Fallot | 13 |
| Heterotaxy | 10 |
| Total anomalous pulmonary venous return | 10 |
| Double outlet right ventricle | 9 |
| *l*-Transposition of the great arteries | 6 |

(254/0.7 = 363) in our geographic region, a daunting undertaking.

Recognizing the theoretical and practical limitations to full fetal ascertainment, what are the lessons that can be derived from the live-born population and applied to the practice of prenatal cardiology? Structural cardiac anomalies that are readily recognized by a fetal echocardiographer can be divided into high and low risk for chromosomal abnormalities, syndromic abnormalities and major organ malformations.

As can be seen in Table 5, atrioventricular septal defects, coarctation of the aorta, double outlet right ventricle/tetralogy of Fallot (for chromosomal abnormality), heterotaxy and cono-truncal abnormality (for both syndromic abnormality and organ malformation) form the high-risk group. On the other hand, chromosomal abnormality was not encountered in this patient population in infants with 'laevo' transposition of the great arteries, tricuspid valve atresia or double inlet left ventricle and was rare with transposition of the great arteries, pulmonary stenosis and pulmonary atresia.

Based on this data, it may be reasonable to defer amniocentesis in the fetus with isolated severe right heart obstruction. But there is evidence that the yield of amniocentesis will still be important in the decision-making process in most other major cardiac abnormalities, particularly across the spectrum of outflow defects.

## OUTCOME OF INFANTS WITH CONGENITAL HEART DISEASE

Factors impacting on the outcome of infants with congenital heart disease relate to timely recognition, accurate diagnosis, appropriate medical management and expert surgical intervention when required. As can be seen in this data set, however, the presence of associated non-cardiac anomalies is also a major determinant of outcome. In some instances, co-existing lethal chromosomal abnormalities take precedence over potentially repairable cardiac defects. In others, multiple organ malformations, while individually manageable, may prove overwhelming. Prematurity and intrauterine growth retardation, seen most frequently in tetralogy of Fallot and double outlet right ventricle, provide additional obstacles to successful outcome.

In trying to extrapolate retrospectively to the fetal cardiac population, it has been my contention that recognition of all of these factors is vital in painting a complete picture for realistic prenatal counseling. It is not unreasonable to expect the fetal outcome to be substantially different from that reported by regional medical centers dealing with a predominantly referred population of infants who, while often having severe cardiac malformations, will also often have an isolated malformation. The dismal outcome reported by large fetal programs, even when elective termination of pregnancy is excluded from the data, bears testimony to this reality[7].

In the BWIS population of 4390 patients, there is a subset of patients diagnosed only by autopsy, live-born infants who died in the community hospital setting without recognition or without the potential benefit of referral. In many respects, these infants appear to be the link to the fetal population. Compared to the 4305 infants clinically diagnosed, this subgroup was more likely to have complex malformations (62% versus 35%), to have major non-cardiac malformations (60% versus 25%) and to weigh less than 1500 g (18% versus 3%). Clearly, this group presents the most difficult management situation.

For the entire case population there was an all-cause mortality of 18%. Case mortality appeared to improve from 25% in 1981–1983 to 14% in 1987–1989. However, as noted in a different context earlier, much of the improvement in survival relates to the influx of infants with minor defects, particularly small ventricular or atrial septal defects and pulmonary valve stenosis. Review of the findings from large subgroups of patients points out the difference between perceived and real improvement in 1-year

**Table 6** Occurrence and mortality from all causes

| Lesion | n | 1981–83 | 1984–86 | 1987–89 |
|---|---|---|---|---|
| Atrioventricular septal defects | 318 | 31% | 30% | 28% |
| Hypoplastic left heart syndrome | 166 | 97% | 85% | 67% |
| Aortic valve stenosis | 127 | 21% | 18% | 17% |
| Coarctation | 200 | 16% | 23% | 13% |
| Ventricular septal defects memb./musc. | 1317 | 7% | 5% | 3% |

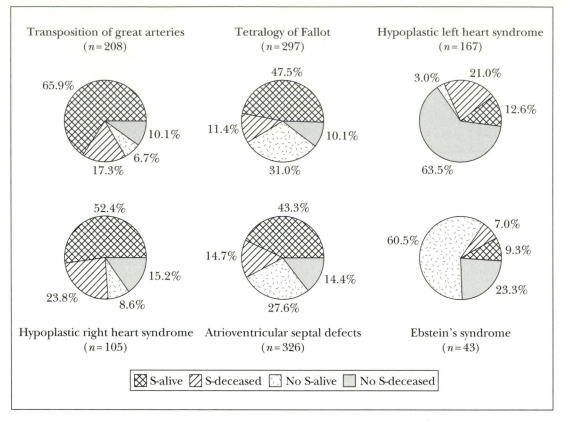

**Figure 3** Outcome in six selected lesions, 1981–1989. Cases segregated by surgery(S) or no surgery (No S), alive or deceased. Awareness of the important role of medical mortality (No S) in counseling is vital

survival (Table 6). Little change is seen over the 9 years for atrioventricular septal defects and coarctation, where full ascertainment was likely to be the rule throughout the time period. A real improvement in survival for infants with hypoplastic left heart syndrome probably represents a philosophical change in management, where offering the staged Norwood procedure or cardiac transplantation became increasingly accepted by physicians and parents in this geographic region during the mid-1980s. Successful application of these interventions was beginning to have an impact on survival by the late 1980s, even as the number of infants with hypoplastic left heart syndrome was decreasing, probably because of prenatal detection and intervention. Once again, improved outcome of the group with ventricular septal defects was influenced by the dispropor-

tionate number of infants with small ventricular septal defects enrolled in the data set in later years.

To highlight the regional experience, Figure 3 depicts the outcome of infants with six selected lesions, all of which we would hope to recognize in prenatal life, given the opportunity. We must recognize the significant medical mortality in infants with tetralogy of Fallot (10.1%), transposition of the great arteries (10.1%), atrioventricular septal defects (14.4%), Ebstein's anomaly (23.3%), hypoplastic left heart syndrome (63.5%) and hypoplastic right heart (15.2%). Medical morbidity and mortality cannot be avoided in the process of parental education and medical planning for optimal perinatal care. Improvements in surgical management may already permit a more optimistic picture than experienced in the 1980s.

## CONCLUSION

Management of the fetus with congenital heart disease will be impacted by continued improvement in technology, permitting more precise prenatal definition of both cardiac and non-cardiac malformations. Successful prenatal intervention and improvements in perinatal medical and surgical management can be expected to enhance neonatal survival. Clearly, the most profound and fundamental change in fetal management will be based on improved understanding of the epidemiologic and genetic information derived from populations such as the BWIS. Successful application of molecular genetic techniques to subsets of infants with specific cardiac and non-cardiac malformation will hopefully soon permit therapies aimed at the prevention of this group of devastating birth defects.

# References

1. Fyler, D. C. (1980). Report of the New England Regional Infant Cardiac Program. *Pediatrics*, **65** (suppl.), 375–461
2. Ferencz, C., Rubin, J. D., Loffredo, C. A. and Magee, C. A. (eds.) (1993) *Perspectives in Pediatric Cardiology Vol 4. Congenital Heart Disease – The Baltimore–Washington Infant Study 1981–1989.* (New York: Futura Publishing Company)
3. Martin, G. R., Perry, L. W. and Ferencz, C. (1989). Increased prevalence of ventricular septal defect: epidemic or improved diagnoses. *Pediatrics*, **83**, 200–3
4. Payne, R. M., Johnson, M. C., Grant, J. W. and Strauss, A. W. (1995). Toward a Molecular Understanding of Congenital Heart Disease. *Circulation*, **91**, 494–504
5. Cook, A. C., Allan, L. D., Anderson, R. M., Sharland, G. and Fagg, N. L. K. (1991) Atrioventricular septal defect in fetal life – a clinicopathological correlation. *Cardiol. Young*, **1**, 334–43
6. Berg, K. A., Boughman, J. A., Ferencz, C. and Clark, E. B. (1987) Estimation of the risk of a chromosomal abnormality in a fetus with echodiagnosed AV canal or type II VSD. *Am. J. Cardiol.*, **60**, 642
7. Smythe, J. F., Copel, J. A. and Kleinman, C. S. (1992) Outcome of prenatally detected cardiac malformations. *Am. J. Cardiol.*, **69**, 1471–4

# Index